GET INTO MEDICAL SCHOOL

600 UKCAT PRACTICE QUESTIONS

Includes Full Mock Exam

Comprehensive tips, techniques & explanations

Olivier Picard, Laetitia Tighlit, Sami Tighlit, David Phillips

1

Published by ISC Medical
Hamilton House, Mabledon Place, London WC1H 9BB
Tel: 0845 226 9487

First Edition: June 2009 reprinted February 2010
ISBN13: 978-1-905812-09-7
A catalogue record for this book is available from the British Library.

The information within this text is intended as a revision aid for the purpose of the UKCAT only. Any information contained within the texts used in the verbal reasoning section should not be regarded as views held by the authors of this book, but simply as text used in a question-setting context with the view of preparing students for a competitive test.

Printed in the United Kingdom by:
Purbrooks Ltd, Gresham Way, Wimbledon Park, London SW19 8ED

INTRODUCTION

The UKCAT (UK Clinical Aptitude Test) is designed to assess a spectrum of skills in candidates to medical and dental schools, ranging from their ability to manipulate data and numbers, to their ability to derive meaningful conclusions from somewhat incomplete or confusing data.

The difficulty in such tests does not rest so much in the actual difficulty of each question independently (ultimately, if given proper time to do the test, everyone would get a fairly high score) but in the fact that candidates only have a few seconds to get it right. It is that added pressure which makes many candidates stress on the day.

As a result, although there is no need to revise any specific material to answer any of the questions, those who have had a maximum amount of practice will fare much better than the others. Not only will they know what to expect from each type of question and will therefore spend less time on the day of the test to get used to the format of the test, they will also have familiarised themselves with all the potential traps that can be laid by the examiners. In addition, by practising intensely, candidates will have learnt valuable techniques that will save them a considerable amount of time on the day.

With over 600 questions spanning 400 pages, this book contains an overwhelming range of exercises that will enable all UKCAT candidates to refine and optimise their technique to answer questions under strict time constraints.

This book replicates the breadth and depth of the different types of questions that can be asked in the live UKCAT. The spectrum of difficulties that it covers (from normal to stretching) makes it an ideal preparation tool for all those who want to achieve a high score and maximise their chances of getting into the medical school of their choice.

Good luck with your preparation!

Olivier, Laetitia, Sami and David

CONTENTS TABLE

INTRODUCTION

TO THE

UKCAT

1 Background

INTRODUCTION

The UKCAT was set up by a group of medical schools with the view of assisting in the selection of candidates for entry into medical and dental school by testing a range of abilities relevant in the context of their degrees and their subsequent professional life.

The testing is computerised and takes place under controlled conditions in each of the 150 testing centres every year, typically between early July and early September. Full details on how the exam is run and the universities to which the test applies can be found each year on the official UKCAT website at www.ukcat.ac.uk.

THE TEST

The test comprises five distinct sections, only four of which actually count for the purpose of entry into the medical or dental school. The five sections are as follows:

Quantitative reasoning
This section tests the candidates' ability to manipulate data and interpret charts, tables and other numerical information in order to resolve problems. This section contains 40 numerical questions which must be answered in a total of 22 minutes (this includes 1 minute to read the instructions). A hand-held calculator is made available to candidates during the exam.

For in-depth explanations, techniques and quantitative reasoning practice exercises, go to page 11.

Abstract reasoning
The abstract reasoning section of the test assesses the candidates' ability to analyse information in an environment where there are distracting features, to derive and test hypotheses, and to query their judgement when needed. This is achieved by asking candidates to identify relationships

between various abstract shapes. This section contains 65 questions which much be answered in 16 minutes (this includes 1 minute to read the instructions).

For in-depth explanations, techniques and abstract reasoning practice exercises, go to page 83.

Verbal reasoning
This section tests the candidates' ability to analyse an important amount of text in order to determine whether specific conclusions can be drawn from the information presented. The test includes 11 pieces of text, each of approximately 200 to 300 words. Each piece of text attracts 4 questions. All 44 resulting questions must be answered in 22 minutes (this includes 1 minute to read the instructions).

For in-depth explanations, techniques and verbal reasoning practice exercises, go to page 143.

Decision analysis
The decision analysis tests the candidates' ability to interpret information and make decisions in situations when not all information is available, or where the information available is not always of the highest quality. This section involves 26 questions all based around the same code. All questions must be answered within 30 minutes (this includes 1 minute to read the instructions).

For in-depth explanations, techniques and verbal reasoning practice exercises, go to page 193.

Non-cognitive analysis
This section of the test (30 minutes maximum) is compulsory for all candidates but it is not used by medical and dental schools to assess the suitability of candidates for selection into the school. In fact, candidates may be asked questions which differ from those asked to other candidates. The purpose of the test is to provide medical and dental schools with information regarding personal attributes not tested by the main four components (such as empathy, integrity, resilience, etc.).

The non-cognitive analysis test consists of a series of questions asking candidates to determine how they would react in given situations. Example questions include asking about how you would react if you knew that one of your friends had cheated during an important examination, or whether you feel that it is always important to take other people's opinions on board when making decisions.

There is nothing that you can do to prepare for this part of the test and, as such, it would be pointless to practise any questions. The best advice that we can give you is that you answer the questions as truthfully as you can using the options given to you at the time.

In fact, candidates who try to second-guess what the examiners "would like to hear" will most likely come across as people who are contradictory or who are giving mixed signals. For this part of the test, honesty is the best policy.

The medical and dental schools which use the UKCAT agree that this section is not suitable for the purpose of selection. As such, results will only be used (if at all) by each school once the candidate has been accepted in order to guide and counsel students during the course of their studies.

SUMMARY TABLE

Test	Number of questions	Time for questions	Time for instructions	Total time
Quantitative Reasoning	40	21 mins	1 min	22 mins
Abstract Reasoning	65	15 mins	1 min	16 mins
Verbal Reasoning	44	21 mins	1 min	22 mins
Decision Analysis	26	29 mins	1 min	30 mins
Non-Cognitive Analysis	varies	30 mins	-	30 mins

2   How the test results are used

MARKING OF THE UKCAT

Each of the sections of the UKCAT is marked separately out of 900. Each university then uses the results communicated to them about their applicants in a way that it sees fit. This means that there is not an official one-size-fits-all pass or fail mark.

The manner in which medical and dental schools use UKCAT results changes every year. In addition, the methods vary from one university to the next. Indeed some universities regard the UKCAT as merely being a small part of an overall recruitment process and use the results as a guide, whilst others have strict criteria and cut-off marks for their applicants.

Here are some examples of the ways in which universities have used the UKCAT results in the past:

- The test results are averaged across all four main sections to give an overall score out of 900. Only applicants with a score above a given cut-off mark are considered. A score of 600 out of 900 has often been used, though some universities have been known to use lower cut off marks, and few universities have been known to use higher cut off marks, as high as 670.

- The results of the four sections are considered separately; candidates are expected to achieve a given cut-off mark in <u>each</u> of the sections (often 600 out of 900).

- Candidates are ranked according to their average UKCAT test results and only those in the top x % (typically top 20%, 25% or 50% depending on the university and the year) are invited to interview.

As you can see, there is a wide variety of ways in which the UKCAT results are being used. Generally speaking, and based on past experience of hundreds of applicants, several universities seem to adopt a cut-off point or at least a reference point of 600 marks out of 900. Candidates should therefore do their best to ensure that they obtain at least two-thirds of the marks available as this will cover a broad range of medical schools. Those applying for the very competitive medical or dental schools should target scores of 700 or over.

WHAT THIS MEANS FOR YOU

The issue of a likely cut-off point being adopted by many universities means two things:

- You must identify your weaker areas and practise questions for the tests which cause you the most trouble so that you maintain a high average score as well as a high individual score for each section.

- You must consider the issue of the mark that you are targeting in relation to the time that you know it takes you to do an exercise within each type of test. For example, if you know that you keep getting your sums wrong when you calculate too quickly, you might want to attempt only 80% of the exercises in the quantitative reasoning test, with the view of getting 90% of the answers to those questions right, instead of rushing through all the questions and ending up getting only 20% of the questions right.

PRACTISE, PRACTISE, PRACTISE

Ultimately, your goal should be to achieve the highest possible score. Worrying unnecessarily about any cut-off point which may or may not exist in such and such a university is a secondary matter when it comes to the actual day of the test.

To help you achieve this, the 600 practice and mock exam questions contained in this book will help you understand the requirements for each of the four main tests and will help you build a range of skills and techniques which will ensure you save a considerable amount of time.

We would recommend that you first attempt the practice questions for each test individually, before moving to the mock exam, which you should, as far as you can, perform in real time.

QUANTITATIVE REASONING

TIPS & TECHNIQUES

+

120
PRACTICE QUESTIONS & ANSWERS

3 Quantitative Reasoning
Format, Purpose & Key Techniques

FORMAT

The quantitative reasoning section of the UKCAT consists of 10 scenarios, each consisting of:

- Numerical data usually provided in the form of graphs or tables, but sometimes as part of a piece of text, and

- Four questions requiring calculations and interpretations to be carried out. For each question, you are provided with five possible answers, from which you must choose the correct one.

To answer all 40 questions (10 scenarios x 4 questions each) you are allocated 22 minutes. This includes 1 minute for reading the generic instructions provided and 21 minutes to answer the 40 questions. Roughly speaking this represents less than 30 seconds per question depending on the complexity of the scenario.

The level of familiarity with numbers is that of a good GCSE pass. A calculator is provided on the day of the exam.

PURPOSE

The quantitative reasoning section of the UKCAT tests your numerical problem-solving abilities and your ability to extract and manipulate information in doing so. As with any other scientific discipline, Medicine requires a large degree of data analysis. This is sometimes based on readily available information, and at other times based on more tenuous information. Whether you are attempting to calculate the dose of a drug that needs to be administered to a patient in relation to their weight, age and other key factors; whether you are designing a new rota for your team to make sure that it is fully compliant with regulations; or whether you are trying to make sense of statistics quoted in a research paper that you are reading, Medicine requires an ability to use information in order to solve problems and therefore requires a degree of mental agility too.

KEY TECHNIQUES

Find a strategy that works for you

The main difficulty of this section is that you only have on average 30 seconds to find the answer to each question. Given that some questions and scenarios can be lengthy to read through, in reality you will probably find that you only have 20 seconds left for each question once you have finished reading everything. Different candidates will handle this matter in different ways and, before making decisions on your own strategy, you may wish to consider the following points (looking at the individual questions rather than the scenarios):

- Although you obviously need to aim for the highest possible score, it would be foolish to try to answer every single question if it means getting most of them wrong simply because you wanted to go quickly. It may be better to attempt 80% of the questions properly and get them all right rather than mess up on 100% of the questions provided because you rushed your calculations.

- The test is not negatively marked (i.e. you don't get penalised explicitly for getting an answer wrong). So, never leave a question unanswered. If you have not managed to come to a sensible answer for a specific question, or if you have run out of time, make sure that you give an answer, even if you have to guess it. Even if you answered randomly you would expect to get it right by chance 20% of the time since you have to pick one option out of five. If you make an educated guess rather than a random guess, the probability of getting it right is even higher. So, if you had to make a guess on, say, 25% of the questions because you did not have time to answer them, you would gain on average an additional score of 5% (20% of 25%). This could well tip you over the threshold of 600 marks that many medical schools seem to regard as a good score.

- You will find that some questions are much easier than others and that these easier questions are littered throughout the test. One strategy is to go through the questions systematically, but picking out the easier ones to ensure that they get done quickly. Once you have done the easier questions then go back to the more difficult questions and address them until you run out of time. This strategy ensures that you do not get held up for prolonged periods of time by some of the more

13

difficult questions and you score as many of the easy points as possible. It does, however, have three drawbacks:

    i.   It requires some practice to identify at a glance whether a question is likely to be an easy, quick question or whether it will take some time to answer. However, with practice, this should be easily resolved. The questions in this book will help you with this.

    ii.   When you go back to a previous difficult question, you have to remind yourself of the context of the question once again.

    iii.   Going back and forth on the computer system may waste time by itself.

- Another strategy is to go through the questions in order and to force yourself to move on to another question once you have overstepped the 30-second target allocated to each question; unless you can see that you are about to get to a result quickly thereafter, in which case you can allow yourself a few more seconds. This has the advantage of not allowing you to get bogged down with the questions which are taking a long time and will also enable you to have a go at most of the questions. However, it presents a serious risk of making you rush for the sake of going through all the questions and of placing quantity over quality.

- A better strategy is to monitor your time carefully and to give yourself some time markers that you can use to determine whether you are on track or not. For example, you should have done the first 5 scenarios in the first 10 minutes. If you are lagging behind then you need to speed up a little. Try not to time each question individually. Not only will you become so obsessed with time that you will actually lose valuable seconds looking at the clock, but you would be ignoring the fact that some scenarios are easier than others and therefore that it is the average of 2 minutes per scenario which counts rather than the timing on each individual scenario.

- If you are getting bogged down with one question and feel that you are not likely to find the answer easily despite your efforts, cut your losses and move on. You may have wasted valuable time but you don't want to waste more through stubbornness if it means losing marks because you did not have time to do other questions. Simply take a guess and move on. You can always go back to it later.

- The strategy you should ultimately adopt will depend on your way of working, your attitude to risk and whether you get stressed or remain composed when facing pressure. Many candidates adopt a halfway strategy whereby they go systematically through every question, give it a shot for, say, 20 seconds and then decide whether it is worth investing more time in it or just taking a guess and moving on. If they have time at the end, they then go back to the answers they guessed and refine their answers as necessary.

Don't study the data in-depth immediately. Scan it intelligently
In some scenarios, the amount of data given could be such that it would take you 2 minutes just to read it all and understand it. In such cases, it will therefore be difficult to assimilate everything and answer the questions in 2 minutes. Rather than read and assimilate the full amount of data given, you may wish to scan through it quickly to understand the "type" of information that you are given. Then, when you read the question, you will be able to determine quickly what sort of data you need to answer it; having glanced at the data before, you will know exactly where to find it when you need it.

Use order of magnitudes whenever possible
Some questions give the choice between answers in a wide range. In some cases, you can actually derive the answer simply by looking at the data and the orders of magnitude of the different answers. For example, consider the following table:

Data set	143	176	129	172

If you were being asked the question: "What is the average of the above numbers", with possible answers being 70, 100, 135, 155 and 170, you could answer quickly that the answer has to be 155 since 70 and 100 are lower than the smallest number in the list, 135 is very close to 129 and has to be too low, and 170 is almost equal to the highest number in the list.

This question could therefore be answered simply by glancing at the data and exercising judgement, without the need for any calculation. In many questions you will obviously be required to carry out some calculations but in many cases you can simplify your task drastically and save yourself a lot of time by identifying suitable shortcuts and narrowing down the scope of the calculations that you need to perform.

This technique will not work when the options are too close together so you will need to learn to recognise when such an approach is possible. Some of the exercises in this book will give you an opportunity to do this and we have provided full explanations in the answers.

When appropriate, start from the options given

In some questions, you may need to write an equation which, although it looks simple, may take a few seconds too many to resolve. Rather than trying to find the answer by resolving the equation from a pure mathematical perspective, which could take some time, simply try the options given and see which one fits. If you have managed to rule out some of the options through pure logical deduction then hopefully you will only have to try a few of the options on display.

Save valuable time by converting as few numbers as you can

Some questions provide numbers in one unit and ask for the result in another unit. For example, you may be given the lengths of two sides of a rectangle in metres, and asked to calculate the surface area in square feet. Rather than converting both lengths into square feet and then multiplying one by the other, it is quicker to calculate the area in square metres and then to convert that number into square feet.

Make full use of the whiteboard, if provided

Some questions may require a simple equation to be set and resolved. Although it will always be a simple one, solving it in your head will often result in a plus or minus sign being misplaced or inverted. In previous years, candidates have had access to a computerised whiteboard in the exam. For the more complex calculations, use it to keep track of your reasoning on the board so that you can easily spot any error you may have made.

Convert numbers the right way round

Candidates in a hurry often get their conversation rates the wrong way round. If the text states that the conversion rate is £1.5 = $2.1 then $100 will be equivalent to 100 / 2.1 x 1.5 = £71.43. This result will obviously appear in the list of options, but so will £140 (which is calculated as 100 x 2.1 / 1.5). It is therefore imperative that you check the units in which the data is expressed, that you check the unit in which the result is required and that you apply conversion rates the right way round.

Round numbers as specified or implied by the question
Some questions will ask you to calculate numbers that one would expect to be integers but which, in a calculation, may come out as decimal.

For example, if you are given a recipe which requires 1.5kg of meat and you are told that the meat can only be purchased in packs of 600g, you would need to buy 3 packs to make the dish, and not 1.5 / 0.6 = 2.5. It may well be that 2.5 and 3 are both options offered to you.

Read the text carefully to determine which one would fit best (e.g. if they ask for the average number of packs required to make the recipe, the answer would be 2.5. If they asked how many packs one particular customer should buy, it would be 3).

Follow the question through
It may sound obvious but reading a question too quickly may cause you to miss valuable terms which will then lead you to calculate the wrong answer.

For example, you may have a scenario about two friends who are travelling using different routes. A question may ask "How many more days than Paul will Peter take to complete the journey?" This will mean computing the two different travelling times and then the difference between the two. In many cases, a rushed candidate may calculate both and forget to subtract one from the other. The two individual journey times are likely to feature in the options; the candidate will find an answer which matches his findings but which does not actually answer the full question posed.

Make sure you read the question carefully since, in most cases, the options will have anticipated your mistake.

Get the percentage increase/decrease the right way round
In some questions, you may be asked for the percentage increase or decrease from one year to the next. Remember that the percentage is calculated in relation to the starting point. For example, if sales in 2007 were £800 and sales in 2008 were £1,000 then the percentage increase between 2007 and 2008 was 25% (i.e. 200/800) and not 20% (i.e. 200/1000). Again, you can be sure that both 20% and 25% will feature in the options provided. In a rush, such a mistake is easy to make.

Practise, practise, practise

Although the level of mathematics that you require to solve each question is relatively simple, the main difficulty lies in the timing. Many of the questions are of a similar nature and, although you don't need to acquire or revise any specific knowledge for the quantitative reasoning test, it is important that you familiarise yourself with the various formats in which the information can be presented, and the various difficulties that you can encounter in your reasoning.

4   Quantitative Reasoning Practice Questions

In this section you will find 120 practice questions (20 scenarios, each containing between 4 and 8 practice questions). This is equivalent to three full exams.

The questions have been carefully chosen to represent the different numerical reasoning approaches and levels of difficulty that you may encounter in the live exam. We have deliberately provided more questions per scenario that you would have at the exam to enhance your learning experience. At the end of the section we have also set out detailed explanations on how the answers can be derived. When relevant, we have provided several possible ways of getting to the answer.

The level of difficulty of the questions in this section varies from quick and easy to more challenging. In order to assist with your preparation, we have identified the harder questions with the following symbol: ** next to the question number (e.g.Q3.5**).

Depending on your way of learning and working, you may decide to answer the questions in real time (in which case you would need to allocate an average of 30 seconds per question, i.e. a scenario with 7 questions should be done in 3.5 minutes) or to approach the questions at your own pace in order to build your awareness of the difficulties that you may encounter. The answers to all questions can be found from page 58 onwards.

Once you have practised answering all 120 questions, you should be ready to confront the mock exam at the back of this book and replicate the actual exam's format (i.e. 10 texts, 4 questions each). You may want to wait until you have practised all sections in this book before going ahead with the mock exam.

QR 1 Practice	Exchange Rate

A bank customer who lives in the UK and travels to the US can pay his way with a range of payment methods whilst abroad.

▶ When in the UK, he can go to a Bureau de Change and exchange Pounds Sterling (£) against US Dollars (US$ or $) in cash.

▶ Whilst in the US, he may wish to pay for purchases directly with his credit card, saving him the hassle of handling cash. If he does need cash during his trip, he can withdraw it from a cash machine (ATM) in the US.

		In the USA		In the UK
		Cash withdrawal (ATM)	Credit card purchases	Buying US$
Bank A	Commission	3.00%	3.50%	1.50%
	Fee	£2	0	£6
Bank B	Commission	2.50%	3%	2.00%
	Fee	£3	£1	£5
Bank C	Commission	2.00%	3.20%	2.50%
	Fee	£4	£1	£4
Bank D	Commission	2.00%	3.30%	2.70%
	Fee	£4	£1.5	£4.50

▶ Exchange rate £1 = US$1.70.

▶ A fee is charged for each transaction.

▶ When a UK bank is given Pounds Sterling to change to US Dollars, it first deducts the fee from the amount tendered and then charges commission on the remaining amount. The remainder is converted into Dollars and given to the client.

▶ When a customer spends or withdraws money in the US, his UK bank calculates the commission on the amount of US Dollars withdrawn or paid, adds the commission to the amount, converts the total to Pounds and charges the amount to the customer's account, together with the fee.

PRACTICE QUESTIONS

Q1.1 A customer travels from the UK to the US and, before his departure, exchanges Pounds Sterling in cash at Bank A to obtain a sum of US$850. How much does he give the bank in Pounds Sterling to achieve this?

    a. £507.50   **b.** £507.61   **c.** £509.61 **d.** £513.50 **e.** £513.61

Q1.2 A customer banking with Bank A spends $3,570 on his credit card. How much should he expect to appear on his bank statement for this transaction?

    a. £2068.97   **b.** £2173.50 **c.** £5979.31 **d.** £6180.03 **e.** £6183.03

Q1.3 A customer of Bank B exchanged £380 against US Dollars in cash before his departure. In the US, he withdrew $780 in cash from an ATM in three separate transactions. How much has he spent in total, expressed in Pounds Sterling?

    a. £850.29   **b.** £853.29   **c.** £856.29 **d.** £859.29 **e.** £862.29

Q1.4 A customer has decided to shop around and wants to find the cheapest bank, given that he wishes to spend $3,400 on his credit card on one single transaction when he gets to the US. Which bank should he choose?

    a. Bank A   **b.** Bank B   **c.** Bank C **d.** Bank D **e.** Any Bank

Q1.5 In the US, a Bank C customer wants to buy a US$2,000 present for his wife. How much cheaper in Pounds will it be to pay for it by withdrawing cash in the US, compared to paying by credit card?

    a. £10.12   **b.** £11.12   **c.** £14.12   **d.** £17.12   **e.** £18.12

Q1.6 Bank C has now decided that, for ATM cash withdrawals only, it will reduce its transaction fee to zero and will increase its commission rate instead. Based on a withdrawal of $2,000, what commission should the bank charge in order for the change to be neutral?

    a. 0.20%   **b.** 0.34%   **c.** 1.66%   **d.** 2.34%   **e.** 3.40%

QR 2 Practice	Amusement Park

This table represents the number of tickets sold by a UK amusement park and the ticket prices for the years 2004 to 2007.

Years	Ticket sales					
	Individual Children		Individual Adults		Groups	
	Low season	High season	Low season	High season	Low season Children	Low season Adults
2004	51,000	27,000	38,000	20,000	15,000	17,000
2005	47,000	24,000	34,000	17,000	12,500	13,500
2006	44,000	24,000	32,000	17,000	12,000	14,300
2007	46,000	21,000	34,000	15,500	11,500	13,400
	Ticket prices					
2004/2005	£3.05	£3.55	£5.10	£6.10	£2.05	£4.05
2006/2007	£3.35	£4.00	£5.35	£6.65	£2.00	£4.00

Notes:
- Group tickets are not available in high season.
- A group is defined as 15 or more adults and children aged over 3.

PRACTICE QUESTIONS

Q2.1 By what percentage did the total income from high season sales increase (or decrease) between 2004 and 2005?

   a. –15.33%   **b.** –13.29%   **c.** +7.24%   **d.** +13.29% **e.** +15.33%

Q2.2 In 2006, what proportion of total income did group ticket sales represent?

   a. 10.34%   **b.** 13.34%   **c.** 15.67%   **d.** 17.57%   **e.** 18.35%

Q2.3 Between 2004 and 2005, all categories suffered a drop in the number of tickets sold. One of the six categories experienced a smaller loss than all others when measured as a percentage of the level of 2004 ticket sales. What is that percentage?

a. 7.84%   **b.** 11.53%   **c.** 22.50%   **d.** 23.23%   **e.** 23.33%

Q2.4 Managers of the amusement park are expecting to sell 17,504 Adult High Season tickets in 2008. By how much should the managers increase the ticket price in 2008 (from 2007 prices) in order to obtain the same income as in 2004 in that category?

a. 4.81%   **b.** 12.90%   **c.** 14.26%   **d.** 15.65%   **e.** 16.54%

Q2.5 Managers of the amusement park are thinking of charging the same price for all individual children, regardless of whether they come in low or high season. What price should the park have been charging for individual children throughout 2007 in order to earn the same income as it did in that year?

a. £3.35   **b.** £3.45   **c.** £3.55   **d.** £3.65   **e.** £4.00

Q2.6 The same group of 15 adults goes to the amusement park every year between 2004 and 2007 (both years included) in low season. What is the total saving made by the group over the four years by buying a group ticket instead of individual tickets?

a. £4.20   **b.** £4.80   **c.** £36.00   **d.** £72.00   **e.** £81.00

Q2.7 In 2007, a large company hired the entire amusement park for a day for its employees and their families. This represented 750 adults and 900 children, on the following terms:

▶ Each child was charged 70% of the group low season tariff for children.
▶ Each adult was charged 50% of the group low season tariff for adults.

What was the total cost for the company for the day?

a. £1,200   **b.** £2,760   **c.** £2,810   **d.** £2,990   **e.** £3,430

QR 3 Practice	The Hunters and the Hunted

A field bordering a forest is being regularly used by hunters to shoot game. Its characteristics are as follows:

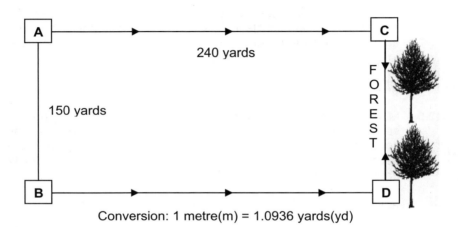

Conversion: 1 metre(m) = 1.0936 yards(yd)

PRACTICE QUESTIONS

Q3.1   What is the area of the field?

   a. 30,101m^2 **b.** 32,919m^2 **c.** 36,000m^2 **d.** 39,370m^2 **e.** 43,055m^2

Q3.2   The field's owner is nearing retirement and wants to share the field between his four sons. He wishes to allocate:

▸ 1/6 of the field to his first son
▸ 2/7 of the field to his second son
▸ 1/5 of the field to his third son
▸ The remainder to his fourth son.

What is the area of the portion of the field allocated to the fourth son?

   a. 12,514yd^2 **b.** 15,895yd^2 **c.** 17,657yd^2 **d.** 18,343yd^2 **e.** 23,486yd^2

Q3.3   Two hunters have killed 14 animals in total (pheasants & rabbits). We are told that:
- Hunter A killed twice as many rabbits as Hunter B
- Hunter A killed three times fewer pheasants than Hunter B
- Hunter A killed 2 pheasants.

How many rabbits did Hunter B kill?

a. 2   **b.** 3   **c.** 4   **d.** 6   **e.** 8

Q3.4   The field's owner wants to use the field to plant potatoes in rows parallel to the AC edge of the field. The first row will be on line AC and the last row will be on line BD. In-between, he will plant one row every 6 inches. Given that there are 36 inches in a yard, how many rows of potatoes will he be able to plant?

a. 900   **b.** 901   **c.** 1440   **d.** 1441   **e.** 5400

Q3.5   The field owner runs along the edge of his field every morning in order to exercise. How long does it take him to run along the full perimeter of the field once, assuming that he runs at a speed of 5 km/h?

a. 5min 35s **b.** 8min 34s **c.** 8min 56s **d.** 9 min 22s **e.** 10min 14s

Q3.6   The field's owner is trying to keep hunters out of the field by installing an electric fence. However, for legal reasons, he can only install the fence one metre inside the field along the entire perimeter. What will be the perimeter of the fence (to the nearest metre)?

a. 705 m   **b.** 706 m   **c.** 709 m   **d.** 713 m   **e.** 714 m

Q3.7   Two hunters walk along the edge of the field, towards the forest. Hunter A walks clockwise from point A. He walks at 60 yd/min. Hunter B walks anticlockwise from point B at a non-specified speed. They meet along the edge of the forest after exactly 5 minutes. At what speed was Hunter B walking?

a. 50 yd/min **b.** 55 yd/min **c.** 56 yd/min **d.** 65 yd/min **e.** 66 yd/min

QR 4 Practice	Diamonds are Forever

Key facts about diamonds:

1. The weight of a diamond is measured in carats. A carat is equivalent to 0.2 grams.
2. The price of rough diamonds is proportionate to the square of the number of carats and is therefore calculated according to the following formula: **Price = (Price of 1 carat) x (Number of carats)^2**
3. The price of a 1-carat diamond varies according to market forces. Currently, a 1-carat rough diamond sells for $125. Hence a 2-carat rough diamond sells for $125 \times 2^2 = \$500$, etc.
4. Diamonds are exported and imported by countries in rough or polished forms.

Diamond import/export figures for Country X for 2008

	Oct – Dec 2008 US$ millions	% change from 2007	Jan – Sep 2008 US$ millions	% change from 2007
Polished Exports	428	- 62.1%	5,812	- 2.2%
Polished Imports	594	- 42.8%	3,787	7.6%
Rough Exports	141	- 73.0%	3,173	11.0%
Rough Imports	315	- 68.1%	4,165	1.7%

PRACTICE QUESTIONS

Q4.1 What is the cost of a rough diamond that weighs 2.6g?

a. $2,275   **b.** $4,225   **c.** $12,653   **d.** $18,845   **e.** $21,125

Q4.2 How much money would a diamond cutter save by buying a 4-carat diamond and a 7-carat diamond, instead of an 11-carat diamond?

a. $7,000   **b.** $9,000   **c.** $8,125   **d.** $9,175   **e.** $12,125

Q4.3 A diamond cutter has purchased a 5-carat rough diamond and must remove half of it in the process of shaping and polishing the rough diamond. He then sells the polished diamond at 20 times the price of a rough diamond of the same weight. How much profit will he make?

a. $12,125　b. $12,500　c.$13,225　d. $14,175　e. $15,625

Q4.4 A diamond cutter has heard rumours that the price of rough diamonds may change soon. He is told that a 4-carat rough diamond might now cost $640. If the new price were to be implemented, what would be the weight of a rough diamond costing $1,960?

a. 4 carats　b. 5 carats　c. 6 carats　d. 7 carats　e. 8 carats

Q4.5 What was the total value of exports in Oct–Dec 2007, to the nearest US$ million?

a. $340m　b. $421m　c. $920m　d. $1,652m　e. $2,117m

Q4.6 By what percentage has the value of polished imports increased or decreased between 2007 and 2008?

a. - 35.2%　b. - 4.04%　c. - 3.88%　d. + 3.88%　e. +4.04

Q4.7 The diamond industry for Country X expects that, for the first quarter of 2009, the net export figure (i.e. the difference between total exports and total imports) will be 20% higher than the average quarterly net export figure over the period Jan–Sep 2008. What is the expected net export figure for the period Jan–Mar 2009 (to the nearest $ million)?

a. $70m　b. $413m　c. $810m　d. $1,033　e. $1,240m

Q4.8 What is the average quarterly income from polished exports in 2008?

a. $428m　b. $1,453m　c. $1,560m　d. $1,937m　e. $3,120m

| QR 5 Practice | **Printing** |

Printing costs
Digital printing (normal quality):
- Initial set-up cost: none
- 6p per page up to total 300,000 pages
- 5p per page between 300,001 pages and 600,000 pages
- 4p per page above 600,001 pages
- The total quantity printed determines the price per page. The same price is charged for all pages, e.g. for 500,000 pages, all pages will be charged at 5p.

Litho printing (higher quality):
- Initial set up cost: £1000
- 6p per page up to total 200,000 pages
- 4.5p per page between 200,001 and 550,000 pages
- 3.5p per page above 550,001 pages
- The total quantity printed determines the price per page. The same price is charged for all pages, e.g. for 300,000 pages, all pages will be charged at 4.5p.

Cover printing
- One colour only:
  - ► £1.50 per book if ordering 1599 books or less
  - ► £1.40 per book if ordering between 1600 and 1999 books
  - ► £1.00 per book if ordering 2000 or more books
- More than one colour: Add 20% to the cost of "one-colour only" printing regardless of the number of colours.

Lamination of the cover
- Matt laminate: 20p per book
- Gloss laminate: 12p per book

Retail data
- Bookshops purchase books directly from the publisher at 75% of the Recommended Retail Price (RRP)

PRACTICE QUESTIONS

Q5.1 Mr Scribbler wants to print 1600 copies of his 126-page book. He wants the book printed using the litho technique, with a cover printed with one colour only and laminated in gloss. How much will it cost?

a. £10,547   **b.** £11,664   **c.** £12,504   **d.** £12,654   **e.** £14,678

Q5.2 A customer needs 3,000 covers, and hesitates between 2 options:
- Option A: 1 colour, matt laminate
- Option B: 2 colours, gloss laminate

How much cheaper is Option A compared to Option B?

a. £ 0   **b.** £ 80   **c.** £360   **d.** £960   **e.** £1,034

Q5.3 A publisher had one of his titles printed at a cost of £34,500. He sold all copies of the book to a bookshop and made a profit of £9,672. The Recommended Retail Price for the book is £16. How many copies of this book did he sell to the bookshop?

a. 2156   **b.** 2761   **c.** 3681   **d.** 4256   **e.** 6783

Q5.4 On 1 January, the publisher asked the printer for a quote based on 2000 copies of a book of 300 pages to be printed using digital technology with a one-colour gloss-laminated cover. On 10 January, he realised the book had, in fact, 400 pages. What is the difference between the actual price paid for the printing of the 400-page books, and the price originally quoted for 300 pages?

a. £1,690   **b.** £2,000   **c.** £4,690   **d.** £8,000   **e.** £10,000

Q5.5 A customer wants 50 copies of a 30-page book printed but cannot afford to pay the full price. The book is to be printed using digital technology and has a three-colour cover which is to be laminated gloss. As a gesture of goodwill, the printer charges him a lower printing cost per page and hands out a total invoice for £156. What price did the printer charge per page?

a. 2p   **b.** 3p   **c.** 4p   **d.** 5p   **e.** 5.5p

QR 6 Practice	Fishy Business

A fish enthusiast buys a fish tank with the following characteristics:

Dimensions
Rectangular base (Length: 2m, Width: 1.50m), Volume: 2,250 litres

Filling the tank with water
In order to avoid excessive pressure on the glass panels of the tank, the fish tank should be filled so that the water level does not go over 80% of its height.

Water treatment
If using tap water, new water added to the tank should be treated with a special solution. Dosage: 1 drop of the solution per litre of water added. The solution is available in bottles of 250ml. Each drop has a volume of 0.05ml.

Fish population
In order to avoid illnesses and stress to the fish population, fish enthusiasts should avoid populating the tank with too many fish. On average there should be no more than 2.5cm of fish per 4.5 litres of water, e.g. a 9-litre tank could take 1 fish of 5cm, 2 fish of 2.5cm each, etc.

PRACTICE QUESTIONS

Q6.1 The fish enthusiast decides to clean the tank before using it by filling it completely with water up to the very top, ignoring the 80% rule. He places the tank under a tap which has a flow rate of 6 litres per minute. How long will it take to fill the tank?

   a. 2h 50min **b.** 4h 10min **c.** 4h 15min **d.** 6h 15min **e.** 6h 25min

Q6.2 The fish enthusiast decides to fill the tank with just water, i.e. no ornaments, gravel or plants, filling it to the maximum level recommended. What volume of water treatment solution will he need to add to the water?

   a. 9 ml   **b.** 90 ml   **c.** 112.5 ml   **d.** 900 ml   **e.** 1125 ml

Q6.3 The fish enthusiast decides to introduce 60 fish into the tank and notices that, once he has done so, the level of the water has risen by 0.5cm. What is the average volume of a fish?

    a. 190 cm^3 **b.** 210 cm^3 **c.** 250cm^3 **d.** 320 cm^3 **e.** 450 cm^3

Q6.4 The fish enthusiast decides to place gravel on the floor of his tank. The gravel occupies 15% of the total volume of the tank. The enthusiast then fills up the tank to the maximum recommended limit. What is the maximum recommended number of fish of 10cm each which the enthusiast will be able to place in the tank?

    a. 81   **b.** 82   **c.** 83   **d.** 84   **e.** 85

Q6.5 The fish enthusiast prefers to tile the bottom of the tank with decorative tiles which are square-shaped and measure 12.5cm on each side. How many tiles will he require?

    a. 72   **b.** 96   **c.** 192   **d.** 194   **e.** 204

Q6.6 The fish enthusiast wants to supplement the tank with a special lighting unit which fits on top of the tank and would add 18% to its height. What is the total height of the combined tank and lighting unit?

    a. 50.75cm   **b.** 75cm   **c.** 88.5cm   **d.** 94.7cm   **e.** 98.6cm

Q6.7 Gravel for the tank can be bought in bags of 5kg. The label on the bag states that the contents of the bag are enough to cover a surface of 1m^2 with a thickness of 7cm of gravel. The fish enthusiast lays down 3cm of gravel at the bottom of the tank, covering the entire surface evenly. What is the weight of the gravel that he has placed into the tank?

    a. 2.1 kg   **b.** 3.9 kg   **c.** 5.0 kg   **d.** 6.4 kg   **e.** 11.7 kg

Q6.8 A tank's price is proportionate to its volume. A cubic tank with edges of 30cm costs £47. How much would the fish enthusiast's tank cost?

    a. £2,350   **b.** £3,133   **c.** £3,917   **d.** £4,549   **e.** £4,551

QR 7 Practice	World News

Number of newspapers sold over Years 1 to 5

	Newspaper A	Newspaper B	Newspaper C
Year 1	130,000	110,000	98,700
Year 2	230,000	140,000	100,000
Year 3	135,000	110,000	190,000
Year 4	136,000	156,000	167,000
Year 5	133,000	176,000	156,000

Newspaper A:
- Sold in New Zealand, Australia and West Africa.
- Price is 70p in all years.

Newspaper B:
- Sold only in Europe.
- Years 1, 2 and 3: Price is 65p.
- Years 4 and 5: Price is 60p.

Newspaper C:
- 37% of copies sold in Europe. 63% of copies sold in Asia.
- Years 1, 2 and 3: Price is 55p in all regions.
- Years 4 and 5: Price is 50p in Europe and 60p in Asia.

PRACTICE QUESTIONS

Q7.1 In Year 1, what proportion of the total number of newspapers sold that year did Newspapers A and C represent?

a. 59%	b. 63%	c. 68%	d. 76%	e. 79%

Q7.2   What was the income for Newspaper C in Year 5?

   a. £86,166   **b.** £86,245   **c.** £87,135   **d.** £87,576   **e.** £87,828

Q7.3   What was the total income for Europe in Year 4?

   a. £91,585   **b.** £110,165   **c.** £111,350   **d.** £124,495   **e.** 134,460

Q7.4   Between Year 5 & Year 6, the <u>number</u> of newspapers sold changed as follows:
   - Newspaper A: sales dropped by 50%
   - Newspaper B: sales increased by 133%
   - Newspaper C: sales increased by 5/9th.
   How many newspapers were sold in Year 6 (nearest thousand)?

   a. 231,000   **b.** 384,000   **c.** 543,000   **d.** 719,000   **e.** 923,000

Q7.5**   In Year 3, the cost of printing Newspaper B was 30p per copy. The cost of printing increases by 10% every year. In what year will the cost of printing become greater than the income generated by the sales of Newspaper B, assuming that the retail price of Newspaper B remains at Year 5 level?

   a. Year 8   **b.** Year 9   **c.** Year 10   **d.** Year 11   **e.** Year 12

Q7.6   What proportion of all newspaper copies were sold in Europe in Year 3?

   a. 16.2%   **b.** 25.3%   **c.** 35.3%   **d.** 41.4%   **e.** 47.4%

Q7.7   What was the average yearly income for Newspaper C over the five years (to the nearest pound)?

   a. £ 66,842   **b.** £ 79,127   **c.** £ 142,340   **d.** £ 253,256   **e.** £ 376,199

QR 8 Practice	D.I.Y.

An architect has drawn up plans for an apartment using a scale of 1:200.

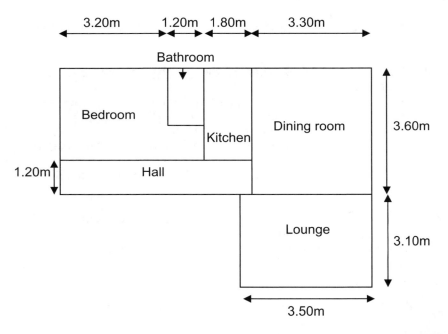

Although the plans only show the surface area at floor level, we know that, in the dining room, there is:

- One French window (1.50m wide and 2m high) on the side opposite to the lounge.
- One door (60cm x 2m) between the hall and the dining room
- One door (90cm x 2m) between the lounge and the dining room

The walls are 2.65m high.

Metre to feet conversion rate: 1m = 3.27ft

PRACTICE QUESTIONS

Q8.1 What is the surface area of the apartment?

    a. 69.68 ft^2 **b.** 181.99 ft^2 **c.** 208.14 ft^2 **d.** 481.72 ft^2 **e.** 680.61 ft^2

Q8.2 What is the surface area occupied by the hall on the architect's plans on paper?

    a. 1.86 cm^2 **b.** 2.84 cm^2 **c.** 3.60 cm^2 **d.** 3.72 cm^2 **e.** 7.44 cm^2

Q8.3 The bedroom has a surface area of 8.76 m^2. What is the length of the longer portion of wall separating the bedroom and the bathroom?

    a. 1.20m   **b.** 1.25m   **c.** 1.30m   **d.** 1.45m   **e.** 1.50m

Q8.4 The landlord wishes to paper over the walls of the dining room. What is the surface covered by the wallpaper?

    a. 13.80 m^2 **b.** 24.80 m^2 **c.** 25.48 m^2 **d.** 30.57 m^2 **e.** 36.57 m^2

Q8.5 What is the total length of the outside walls of the apartment?

    a. 26.2m   **b.** 29.3m   **c.** 32.4m   **d.** 35.4m   **e.** 35.7m

Q8.6 The landlord is contemplating laying down a wooden floor in the lounge. Wooden floors come in planks of 1m length and 10cm width. The planks are laid one after the other in a row; the last plank of a row can be cut easily to fit the dimensions of the room. The part which was cut out can then be used to start the next row. There are no gaps between planks. Planks are sold in packs of 25, with one pack costing £27.53. How much will the owner need to spend to buy the required number of packs?

    a. £119.48 **b.** £137.65 **c.** £143.46 **d.** £164.78 **e.** £166.34

| QR 9 Practice | Going for a Ride |

The following graph shows distances between 8 towns names A to H. Travel between towns is always done using the shortest route.

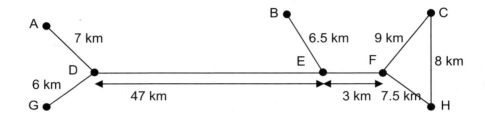

PRACTICE QUESTIONS

Q9.1 It takes 20 minutes for a car to travel from Town E to Town C using the shortest route. How long will the car take to travel from town E to town H using the most direct route, assuming that it goes at the same average speed?

a. 17min 30s b. 17min 40s c. 17min 50s d. 18min 10s e. 18min 20s

Q9.2 A cyclist can ride along the following route: D – E – F – C – H – F – E – B in 10 hours and 30 minutes. What is his average speed?

a. 7.1 km/h b. 7.6 km/h c. 8.0 km/h d. 8.2 km/h e. 8.4km/h

Q9.3 Mr Smith works in Town G. He has 2 hours and 25 minutes free. He decides to go for a ride in his car. He calculates that he has just enough time to go to a certain town, stay there for 49 minutes and get back to work. Which town does he intend to visit, assuming that he drives at an average speed of 70 km/h?

a. Town B b. Town C c. Town E d. Town F e. Town H

Q9.4 A cyclist starts riding from Town C at an average speed of 18 km/h and arrives at his destination 40 minutes later. What is his destination?

a. Town B   **b.** Town D   **c.** Town E   **d.** Town F   **e.** Town H

Q9.5 A cyclist rides from Town D to Town H along the road D-E-F-H. He calculates that if he could ride at a certain average speed, he would arrive into Town H 15 minutes earlier than if he was travelling at 18.4 km/h. What is that speed?

a. 5 km/h   **b.** 10 km/h   **c.** 15 km/h   **d.** 20 km/h   **e.** 25 km/h

Q9.6 As well as a road network, the towns are linked by a tube network which runs exactly underneath the roads. The tube stations are where the dots are shown on the map.

Two passengers leave Town C at the same time to go to Town G, using the route C-F-E-D-G. One passenger travels by tube (no changes necessary) and the other one by car. Between stations, the tube drives at 30 km/h, stopping at each intermediary station for exactly 1 minute. On the road, the car driver drives at 94km/h between D and E, and at 72 km/h on all other roads. How much later than the car driver will the tube passenger arrive in Town G?

a. 45 min   **b.** 59 min   **c.** 1h 28min   **d.** 1h 47min   **e.** 2h 13min

Q9.7 The local authorities have organised a bus services as follows:

- Line FCH: the bus goes in a loop from Town F to Town C to Town H to Town F and so on at 49 km/h (including stops).

- The bus starts at 5am from Point F and stops running at 11pm.

During a one-day shift, how many times will the bus have driven through Town C?

a. 12 times   **b.** 18 times   **c.** 36 times   **d.** 48 times   **e.** 54 times

QR 10 Practice	Hot Chocolate

A chocolate lover purchases a 360g box of powdered drinking chocolate. The label states the following:

NUTRITIONAL INFORMATION			INSTRUCTIONS
	Per 100g (dry powder)	Per 18g serving (with 200ml whole milk)	Put 3 heaped teaspoons (18g) into a mug. Add 200ml of hot milk and stir well. Sit back and relax! For a diet drink, you can use semi-skimmed or skimmed milk. Semi-skimmed milk contains 1.7g of fat per 100ml. Skimmed milk contains 0.3g of fat per 100ml.
Energy (kJ)	1555	845	
KCal	372	200	
Protein (g)	8.9	8.0	
Carbohydrate (g)	65.2	20.4	
Fat (g)	8.4	9.6	

PRACTICE QUESTIONS

Q10.1 How much fat is contained in 200ml of whole milk (to the nearest 0.1g)?

    a. 1.2g   **b.** 3.4g   **c.** 6.8g   **d.** 8.1g   **e.** 9.6g

Q10.2 The customer finds whole milk a bit rich and decides to use a mix of semi-skimmed milk and water instead. He then adds 200ml of the mixed liquid to 18g of powdered chocolate. The total fat content of the resulting drink is 2.464g. Given that water does not contain any fat, what volume of semi-skimmed milk did he use?

    a. 56.0ml   **b.** 81.5ml   **c.** 144.9ml   **d.** 118.5ml   **e.** 170.4ml

Q10.3 The customer uses up the whole box of powdered chocolate, making hot drinks according to the instructions. How many pints of milk will he have used (1 pint = 570ml)?

a. 0.35   **b.** 4.4   **c.** 7.0   **d.** 14.1   **e.** 20.0

Q10.4 The customer is on a diet and, in an effort to reduce his weight, he decides to limit the total daily calories that he gets from the chocolate drink to a strict maximum of 800 kCal. To achieve his objective, he decides to make three chocolate drinks per day using water only (water does not contain any calories) and to make any other chocolate drink using his usual whole milk.

What is the maximum number of whole-milk-based chocolate drinks that he can have in addition to his three daily water-based drinks in order not to breach his resolution?

a. 0 drink   **b.** 1 drink   **c.** 2 drinks   **d.** 3 drinks   **e.** 4 drinks

Q10.5 The customer buys semi-skimmed milk with a label that states that its protein content is 3.3g per 100ml. What is the total amount of protein that he will have drunk once he has made drinks with the entire box of chocolate using standard proportions and semi-skimmed milk instead of whole milk (to the nearest gram)?

a. 66g   **b.** 160g   **c.** 164g   **d.** 244g   **e.** 272g

Q10.6 The calorific value of food is measured in kCal and is calculated by adding the calorific values of protein, carbohydrate and fat. The calorific value of 1g of protein is 4 kCal and the calorific value of 1g of carbohydrate is 4 kCal.

What is the calorific value of 1g of fat, to the nearest gram?

a. 4 kCal   **b.** 6 kCal   **c.** 9 kCal   **d.** 21 kCal   **e.** 44 kCal

QR 11 Practice	Time Traveller

A traveller is looking at a variety of options to travel. All possible connections are shown on the diagram below and can be made by plane.

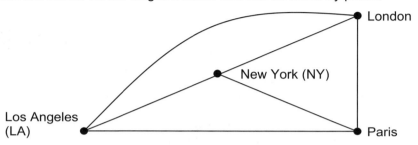

The timetables for the various flights are as follows (all times expressed in local times):

	London to Paris	London to NY	Paris to NY	Paris to LA	NY to LA	London to LA
Departs:	7:50	7:25	6:15	11:15	11:30	10:15
Arrives:	10:15	10:25	8:15	13:25	14:50	13:20
Departs:	9:25	9:10	8:55	13:00	15:50	12:00
Arrives:	11:50	12:10	10:55	15:10	19:10	15:05
Departs:	10:30	11:45	13:20	16:10	17:20	15:10
Arrives:	12:55	14:45	15:20	18:20	20:40	18:15
Departs:	12:25	13:55	15:40	19:45	20:10	18:15
Arrives:	14:50	16:55	17:40	21:55	23:30	21:20

In addition, the traveller is aware that when it is 12 noon in London, the time in:
- Paris is 1pm
- New York is 7am
- Los Angeles 4am

PRACTICE QUESTIONS

Q11.1 What is the duration of a flight from NY to LA?

   a. 20 min   **b.** 2h 20min   **c.** 3h 30 min **d.** 5h 20min   **e.** 6h 20 min

Q11.2 A client wants to travel along the route London → Paris → Los Angeles. He takes the first plane of the day from London and then transfers to the next plane available whenever he reaches a new destination. How much time will have elapsed between his departure from London and his arrival in Los Angeles?

   a. 5h35min   **b.** 12h35min **c.** 13h35min **d.** 14h35min **e.** 15h35min

Q11.3 The plane from Paris to New York flies at an average speed of 730 km/h. What is the distance between the two airports?

   a. 1,460km   **b.** 2,920km   **c.** 4,380km   **d.** 5,840km   **e.** 7,300km

Q11.4 Jack and John want to travel from London to Los Angeles. Jack decides to fly via Paris, whilst John decides to fly via New York. It is 9am and they decide to take the first plane available to them. On arrival at their intermediate destination (Paris or New York), they jump on the first available plane to Los Angeles. When they meet up in Los Angeles, they compare the time it took them to travel from the moment their first plane left to the time their second plane arrived. What is the difference between their respective times?

   a. 1h 55min **b.** 2h 35min   **c.** 2h 45min   **d.** 3h 35min   **e.** 4h 15min

Q11.5 The airline wants to introduce a new flight from Paris to New York such that the flight should arrive in New York 30 minutes before the last flight from New York to Los Angeles departs. At what time should this new flight leave Paris (expressed in local Paris time)?

   a. 11:40   **b.** 13:40   **c.** 15:40   **d.** 17:40   **e.** 19:40

Q11.6 A plane travels on average at 730 km/h and consumes on average 2.1 litres of fuel per kilometre flown. How much fuel does the airline use in 1 day for the Paris to Los Angeles flights?

   a. 3,321   **b.** 13,286   **c.** 17,119   **d.** 68,474   **e.** 75,486

QR 12 Practice	Conferencing & Banqueting

A company specialising in organising conferences has a choice between two different types of contract at one venue.

- A **Daily Delegate Rate (DDR)** contract, whereby they pay a fixed price per delegate which entitles them to a comprehensive range of services (e.g. use of the room, flipchart, water, tea and coffee, lunch, etc.).

- A **Room-Basis (RB)** contract, whereby each services used is charged individually.

The company has collected a brochure from a potential conference venue, which provides the following tariffs information:

The Red Rag Conference Centre	
DDR contract	**RB contract**
£45 per participant (weekend) £50 per participant (weekdays) Includes: - Use of conference room - Projector - Flipchart - 3 tea/coffee breaks - Sit-down lunch - Orange juice at lunch time (1 jug for 5 people) - 1 bottle of water per person NOTE Minimum of 8 participants applies. If the number of participants is less than 8, the fee will be charged for 8 people.	Room hire: - £250 (weekend) - £350 (weekdays) Facilities (per room): - Projector: £189 - Flipchart: £15 Refreshments / Food: - Coffee break: £2.50 per break per person - Orange juice: £10 per jug (serves 5 people) - Sit-down lunch: £20 per person - Buffet lunch: £17 per person - Water: £5 per bottle No minimum requirement on the number of participants applies.

All prices quoted above include VAT on all items.

PRACTICE QUESTIONS

Q12.1 What is the cost for 7 participants on a DDR contract on a Monday?

a. £315   **b.** £350   **c.** £360   **d.** £400   **e.** £450

Q12.2 How much would it cost on the RB contract to replicate the package of services provided under the DDR package for 10 participants on a Sunday?

a. £450   **b.** £500   **c.** £650   **d.** £799   **e.** £817

Q12.3** The company needs the following for a Saturday conference:
- Room
- Flipchart
- 3 servings of tea and coffee
- Sit-down lunch

They are hesitating between the RB rate and the DDR rate (they don't mind getting more than they require if the price is cheaper). For which number of participants would the total DDR cost be greater than the RB cost?

a. 10   **b.** 13   **c.** 14   **d.** 15   **e.** 16

Q12.4 All costs quoted include VAT at 17.5%. The government decides to reduce the VAT rate to 15% for the foreseeable future and the hotel wishes to alter its rates accordingly. What is the new weekend DDR rate after allowance has been made for the new 15% VAT rate?

a. £38.30   **b.** £39.13   **c.** £44.04   **d.** £45.98   **e.** £46.74

Q12.5 The company organises a conference for 50 participants on a Monday, hiring a room by itself and using their own caterer, which charges £30 per person. To authorise the customer to use their own caterer, the hotel adds a surcharge of 12% on the room hire cost. What is the average cost per person?

a. £30.00   **b.** £32.67   **c.** £35.00   **d.** £37.84   **e.** £40.00

QR 13 Practice	Milking It

A farmer owns 15 cows. Each cow produces an average of 8.75 litres of milk per day. He sells his milk to a local cooperative at 33p per kilo. Once milk has been obtained from a cow, 15% of its weight can be extracted to obtain cream. 25% of the weight of the extracted cream represents butter.

1 litre of milk weighs 1.034kg. 1 litre of water weighs 1kg.

PRACTICE QUESTIONS

Q13.1 What weight of butter can the farmer extract on average every day?

    a. 4.921 kg **b.** 4.967 kg **c.** 5.021 kg **d.** 5.089 kg **e.** 5.124 kg

Q13.2 In April, the farmer sold his entire milk production to the same co-operative. How much did he earn?

    a. £1,299.37 **b.** £1,342.68 **c.** £1,343.55 **d.** £1,364.56 **e.** £1,388.34

Q13.3 With a view to inflate his profit, the farmer engages in the dishonest activity of adding water to his milk. The volume of water added is 25% of the volume of raw milk. How much does 1 litre of the new mixture weigh?

    a. 1.000 kg **b.** 1.025 kg **c.** 1.027kg **d.** 1.200kg **e.** 1.250 kg

Q13.4 During the 160 days that the winter season lasts, the farmer requires 19,800kg of hay to feed his 15 cows. He has purchased all the hay required before winter started. After 42 days of winter, the farmer decides to purchase 3 new cows. What additional quantity of hay will he require to feed all the cows for the remainder of the winter period if he wishes each cow to be fed on average the same as each was consuming before the purchase?

    a. 1,039.5kg **b.** 2,135.0kg **c.** 2,920.5kg **d.** 3,052.0kg **e.** 3,960.0kg

QR 14 Practice	A Colourful Life

A paint shop allows its customers to produce any paint colour they like from the three primary colours: red, blue and yellow. Its most popular colours are made by mixing as follows:

Colour	% of Red	% of Blue	% of Yellow
Chocolate	33%	33%	34%
Amazon	10%	80%	10%
Rosebud	50%	45%	5%
Violet	40%	40%	20%
Crimson	70%	20%	10%

PRACTICE QUESTIONS

Q14.1 What volume of yellow paint do 2 litres of Amazon paint contain?

a. 100ml   **b.** 200ml   **c.** 300ml   **d.** 500ml   **e.** 800ml

Q14.2 The shop owner mixes 100ml of Crimson with 400 ml of Amazon. What proportion of red paint does the resulting colour contain?

a. 10%   **b.** 12%   **c.** 22%   **d.** 40%   **e.** 70%

Q14.3 The shop owner has a 1-litre pot of Violet. He wants to add yellow to it in order to obtain Chocolate. Once the yellow paint has been added, what will be the total quantity of Chocolate paint obtained (in litres)?

a. 0.212   **b.** 0.412   **c.** 0.812   **d.** 1.2   **e.** 1.212

Q14.4 An eccentric customer wants to invent a new paint colour obtained by mixing all five mixed colours (i.e. Chocolate, Amazon, Rosebud, Violet and Crimson) in equal quantities. What proportion of blue paint would the resulting colour contain?

a. 15%   **b.** 21.8%   **c.** 43.6%   **d.** 60.3%   **e.** 70.8%

QR 15
Practice

Advertising Rates

A magazine offers businesses an opportunity to purchase advertising space in its pages. The cost of adverts is linked to the number of columns which they span and their height measured in centimetres. The data and rates available are as follows:

Page sizes
- Width: 4 columns
- Height: 28 cm

Advertising rates
- Single column: £50 per cm
- Double column: £75 per cm
- Spanning four columns: £150 per cm
- Advert sizes must be measured in exact number of columns by a whole number of centimetres, i.e. one cannot have an advert measuring 1.5 columns by 3.5 cm
- Minimum height of advert charged for: 3 cm (all adverts of less than 3 cm will be charged as if they had a height of 3 cm)

Add-on for colour
- Black and white: No additional cost
- Full colour: Add 20%

Packages available
- Quarter-page: £1,000 black and white, +20% for colour
- Half-page (vertical or horizontal): £2,000 black and white, +20% for colour
- Full-page: £3,800 black and white, +20% for colour

PRACTICE QUESTIONS

Q15.1 A customer wants to place a full colour advert across two columns, which is 8 cm tall. What will the cost be?

   a. £400   **b.** £480   **c.** £600   **d.** £720   **e.** £800

Q15.2 A customer wants to place a black and white advert across four columns which is 7 cm tall. How much is the cheapest possible option?

a. £900   **b.** £950   **c.** £1,000   **d.** £1,050   **e.** £1,400

Q15.3 Consider the following two scenarios:

Scenario 1
The magazine sells one page of advertising to a lot of small customers who all take out black and white single column adverts. All adverts are more than 3 cm long and are laid out one after the other and side by side without any space between them. The page is completely full, i.e. there is no space left.

Scenario 2:
The magazine sells one page of advertising to a single customer who takes out a full-page black and white advert.

What is the loss of revenue incurred by the magazine if it chooses Scenario 2 instead of Scenario 1?

a. £400   **b.** £1,800   **c.** £2,800   **d.** £3,800   **e.** £5,600

Q15.4 The magazine sells the following adverts:
- 1 full colour quarter page advert
- 1 double column advert (5 cm) – black and white
- 3 single column advert (4 cm) – black and white
- 1 single column advert (2 cm) – black and white

What is the total income made from these sales?

a. £1,850   **b.** £1,875   **c.** £2,125   **d.** £2,275   **e.** £2,325

Q15.5 What is the maximum income that the magazine can derive from one page of advertising?

a. £3,800   **b.** £4,560   **c.** £6,720   **d.** £10,080   **e.** £20,160

QR 16 Practice	A Matter of Time

Recently published statistics show that, on some lines, trains run more slowly than 20 years ago.

The average journey times for three major lines were as follows:

Table showing average journey times in minutes

Journey	1987	2008
CANTERBURY EAST TO LONDON (VICTORIA)		
Canterbury East to Faversham (12 miles)	13	17
Faversham to Chatham (18 miles)	25	25
Chatham to Victoria (34 miles)	43	44
LEWES TO LONDON (VICTORIA)		
Lewes to Haywards Heath	15	20
Haywards Heath to Gatwick	13	14
Gatwick to East Croydon	17	17
East Croydon to Victoria	16	16
SOUTHEND TO LONDON (FENCHURCH STREET)		
Southend to Upminster	28	30
Upminster to Barking	9	8
Barking to Fenchurch Street	12	16

Source for timing: Thomas Cook European Timetables

Note: 1 mile = 1.6093 km

For the purpose of this exercise, you should assume that none of the trains stopped at any of the intermediary stations shown in the table above, i.e. assume that all trains ran non-stop from their city of origin to London.

PRACTICE QUESTIONS

Q16.1 How much longer did the Lewes to London Victoria journey take in 2008 as compared to 1987?

a. 5 min   **b.** 6 min   **c.** 25 min   **d.** 61 min   **e.** 66 min

Q16.2 What was the average speed of the Canterbury East to London Victoria train in 1987 over the whole line (to the nearest km/h)?

a. 47 km/h   **b.** 58 km/h   **c.** 65 km/h   **d.** 76 km/h   **e.** 81 km/h

Q16.3 By what proportion did the journey time increase between Southend and London Fenchurch Street between 1987 and 2008?

a. 9.00%   **b.** 9.26%   **c.** 10.00%   **d.** 10.20%   **e.** 10.26%

Q16.4 The train company's executives think that, in future, they can make the Canterbury East to London Victoria train journey as short as it used to be in 1987 by allowing their trains to run faster on the Faversham to Chatham portion of the route (with the times for the other two portions of the route remaining at 2008 levels).

At what speed would the train need to run on the Faversham to Chatham portion in order for the whole journey to last the same amount of time as in 1987?

a. 43.2 km/h   **b.** 54.0 km/h   **c.** 69.5 km/h   **d.** 86.9 km/h   **e.** 89.6 km/h

Q16.5 The price of a Canterbury East to London Victoria ticket is £15.90. We are told that the price of a ticket on the Lewes to Victoria line is, on a pound per mile basis, the same as a Canterbury East to London Victoria ticket. Given that a ticket on the Lewes to London Victoria line costs £12.40, what is the distance between Lewes and London Victoria (to the nearest mile)?

a. 50 miles   **b.** 55 miles   **c.** 61 miles   **d.** 66 miles   **e.** 82 miles

QR 17
Practice

Within Shopping Distance

A local authority has carried out a survey of the number of shops present within its boundaries. The data consists of the number of shops and the average turnover (in thousands of pounds) plotted against the distance from the county's central town.

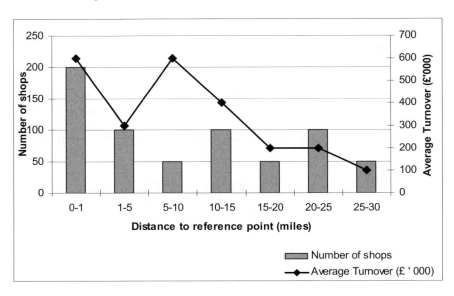

PRACTICE QUESTIONS

Q17.1 How many shops were counted in total by the local authority?

  a. 450　　　**b.** 550　　　**c.** 600　　　**d.** 650　　　**e.** 700

Q17.2 What is the total turnover of the shops located within a distance of 5 miles from the reference point?

  a. £30,000　　**b.** £120,000　**c.** £150,000　**d.** £30m　　**e.** £150m

Q17.3 Which part of the county has the highest total turnover?

a. 0-1   **b.** 1-5   **c.** 5-10   **d.** 10-15   **e.** 20-25

Q17.4 What proportion of total turnover is held by the shops within a 10-mile radius from the reference point?

a. 11.8%   **b.** 33.3%   **c.** 53.8%   **d.** 67.5%   **e.** 70.6%

Q17.5** In the zone within 1 mile of the reference point, all shops must pay a business tax based on their turnover. The business tax is calculated as follows:

- 0.5% payable on the part of turnover up to £100,000
- 1% payable on the part of turnover above £100,000

Assuming that all shops within the zone have a turnover which is greater than £100,000, what is the average amount of tax collected per shop within the zone.

a. £5,500   **b.** £6,000   **c.** £6,500   **d.** £7,500   **e.** £8,000

Q17.6 The council estimates that, with the recession, 20% of shops within a radius of 10 miles will close down whilst the number of shops beyond 10 miles will increase by 5%. What will be the number of shops left standing once the changes have taken effect?

a. 300   **b.** 350   **c.** 595   **d.** 607   **e.** 650

Q17.7 A pensioner lives 12.5 miles away from the reference point. He can only drive a maximum of 7.5 miles in any direction. Assuming that all roads are straight lines and all shops are along those straight roads, how many shops can this pensioner visit?

a. 100   **b.** 150   **c.** 200   **d.** 325   **e.** Can't tell

QR 18 Practice	Shaken, not Stirred

A local bar offers the following cocktails (all quantities expressed in ml):

	Tequila	Cointreau	Lemon Juice	Orange Juice	Vodka	White Rum	Vermouth	Gin
Tequila Sunrise	50			100				
Journalist		5	5				25	50
Screwdriver				50	50			
Balalaika		25	25		25			
Martini							25	50
XYZ		25	25			40		
Vodkatini					50		25	
Velocity							50	25
Orange Bloom		25					25	50
Long Island	25		25		25	25		25

Pure alcohol content for each drink	
Drink	**% of pure alcohol**
Tequila	38%
Cointreau	40%
Lemon Juice / Orange Juice	0%
Vodka	45%
White Rum	40%
Vermouth	15%
Gin	43%

PRACTICE QUESTIONS

Q18.1 What volume of vodka is required to make the following cocktails?

- 2 Screwdrivers
- 5 Balalaika
- 1 Long Island

a. 100ml   **b.** 150ml   **c.** 200ml   **d.** 250ml   **e.** 300ml

Q18.2 What is the volume of pure alcohol contained within one Orange Bloom cocktail?

a. 35.00ml   **b.** 35.25ml   **c.** 35.50ml   **d.** 35.75ml   **e.** 36.00ml

Q18.3 At the start of the night the barman realises that he only has 4 litres of orange juice at his disposal, all of which gets used during the night. The bar till shows that during that night only 8 Tequila Sunrise cocktails have been sold and that no one was served orange juice on its own. How many Screwdrivers were sold that night?

a. 32   **b.** 48   **c.** 56   **d.** 64   **e.** 72

Q18.4 Out of the five following cocktails, which one contains the smallest volume of alcohol?

a. Martini **b.** Vodkatini **c.** Velocity **d.** Orange Bloom **e.** Journalist

Q18.5 Jane normally drinks one Balalaika at the start of the evening. Having got bored with it, she decides today to have an XYZ instead. What is the proportionate change in the volume of pure alcohol that she will consume when she switches to this new cocktail?

a. −42.2%   **b.** −22.4%   **c.** +15.0%   **d.** +22.4%   **e.** +42.2%

Q18.6 During Happy Hour, the bar serves drinks in pitchers (jugs) of 1.5 litres. A group orders the following:

- 2 pitchers of Velocity
- 1 pitcher of Long Island

What volume of Gin is required to make these?

a. 1.15 litres **b.** 1.3 litres   **c.** 1.5 litres   **d.** 2.3 litres   **e.** 4.1 litres

QR 19 Practice	Entente Cordiale

A courier needs to drive from London to Paris and back to deliver a package. The following diagram sets out the route, together with the availability of petrol stations, including prices and distances between each.

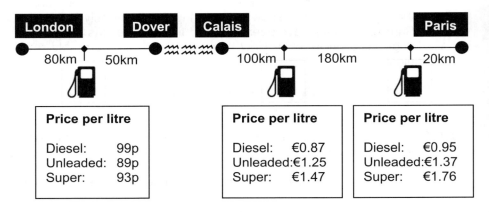

Between Calais and Dover, the car is loaded onto a ferry boat. The cost of a single ferry journey is £75. Including loading and offloading time, the ferry journey takes 2 hours each way.

Exchange rate: £1.00 = €1.20.
Capacity of the car's fuel tank: 45 litres.
The car runs on unleaded petrol.
1 litre of petrol enables the car to drive for 10 km.

PRACTICE QUESTIONS

Q19.1 If the courier drives at an average speed of 110km/h between London and Dover and at an average speed of 120km/h between Calais and Paris, how long will it take him to travel from London to Paris, assuming that he does not stop at any petrol station?

a. 3h 41 min **b.** 3h 49min **c.** 4h 41 min **d.** 5h 41min **e.** 5h 49min

Q19.2 The driver sets out from London with a full tank of fuel. He heads towards Paris with the intention of turning back as soon as he has delivered the package. He forgets to check his fuel gauge and runs out of petrol. At what distance from Paris will he stop?

a. 10km   **b.** 20km   **c.** 30km   **d.** 50km   **e.** 70km

Q19.3 The courier sets out from London with 20 litres of fuel in his tank. He fills his tank to full capacity every time he meets a petrol station and keeps the receipts to give to his boss. How much will his fuel receipts total for the single journey London to Paris?

a. £43.29   **b.** £65.54   **c.** £72.78   **d.** £75.36   **e.** £81.76

Q19.4 The courier's car breaks down in Paris and he is offered a choice between two replacement cars for his return journey to London:

▪ Car A runs on diesel, using 1 litre of diesel per 15km.
▪ Car B runs on super, using 1 litre of super per 10km.

The driver leaves on a full tank (45 litres for both cars) and decides to refuel to full capacity at every petrol station. What is the difference in fuel spend between the two options?

a. €22.05   **b.** €23.13   **c.** €24.21   **d.** €25.03   **e.** €26.05

Q19.5 The courier sets out from London in his usual car on a full tank of unleaded. On the way he stops at a petrol station to fill his fuel tank completely. The refuelling costs him €28.75 (or Pound Sterling equivalent). How many litres of unleaded did he buy?

a. 8 litres   **b.** 23 litres   **c.** 25 litres   **d.** 27 litres   **e.** 41 litres

QR 20 Practice	Parking

A parking meter displays the following information:

PARKING FEES
This car park uses three separate charging time zones

Time Zone 1: Monday – Friday
9:00am – 1:00pm: 20p for each period of 10 minutes
1:00pm – 6:00pm: 30p for each period of 10 minutes

Time Zone 2: Saturday, Sunday & Bank Holiday
9:00am – 6:00 pm: 15p for each period of 20 minutes

Time Zone 3: 6:00pm – 9:00am any day
£1 standard fee regardless of the duration

IMPORTANT NOTES:

1 – Payment is made just as you exit the car park.

2 – Any period started should be paid for in full. For example, a driver staying in the car park for 15 minutes on a Monday afternoon should pay for a full 20 minutes (i.e. 2 x 10-minute periods)

3 – If a car is parked in the car park over several charging zones then a calculation will be made separately for each zone, each being subject to its own minimum charge. For example, a driver arriving at 12:59pm on a Monday and staying 20 minutes will be charged 20p for the period 12:59pm to 1:00pm and 60p for the period 1:00pm to 1:19pm, a total of 80p.

PRACTICE QUESTIONS

Q20.1 A driver arrives at the car park at 9am on a Monday and stays in the car park for 37 minutes. How much will he be charged?

    a. 20p   **b.** 50p   **c.** 74p   **d.** 80p   **e.** £1

Q20.2 A driver enters the car park at 5:55pm on a Monday afternoon and leaves the car park at 6:15pm. How much will he be charged?

a. 40p   **b.** 60p   **c.** £1   **d.** £1.15   **e.** £1.30

Q20.3 A driver parks his car on Monday morning at 9:00am and leaves it in the car park until Sunday evening 6:00pm. How much will it cost him?

a. £59.10   **b.** £65.10   **c.** £71.10   **d.** £77.10   **e.** £83.10

Q20.4 A driver uses the car park all year round and contacts the council to obtain a weekly season ticket. The season ticket he requires is for commuters and only allows him to use the car park Monday to Friday between 8:30am and 6:00pm The cost of the weekly season ticket is £54. How much money will he save in comparison to paying full price for that period?

a. £5   **b.** £10   **c.** £15   **d.** £20   **e.** £25

Q20.5 A driver comes into the car park at 12:58pm and leaves 4 minutes later at 1:02pm on a Monday lunch time after having dropped off his wife at the station. How much will he be charged?

a. 10p   **b.** 20p   **c.** 30p   **d.** 40p   **e.** 50p

Q20.6 A driver only has £4.90 in his pocket to pay for car park fees. He enters the car park on Friday afternoon at 5pm. Until when can he stay in the car park?

a. Friday 9:00pm
b. Saturday 9:00am
c. Saturday 11:00am
d. Saturday 11:40am
e. Saturday 1:40pm

5 Quantitative Reasoning Answers to Practice Questions

QR 1 – Exchange Rate

Q1.1 – e: £513.61

The currency exchange takes place in the UK bank, for which we are instructed that we should take the fee out of the Pound amount and then deduct the commission. Therefore the equation that we need to solve, with X representing the amount in Pounds he needs to pay, is:

$850 =$ (X - £6)   x   (1 - 0.015)   x   1.7
        Deduct fee   Commission   Conversion

This gives X = 850 / 0.985 / 1.7 + 6 = £513.61.

Note that the commission should be calculated as 0.985 of the Pound amount and not the amount divided by 1.015. If I have a sum of £100 on which I need to pay 1.5% commission, I will be left with £98.50 and not with 100/1.015 = £98.52.

Q1.2 – b: 2173.50

This is a similar calculation but this time from the US point of view. From the information given, the amount that should appear on his statement is calculated as follows, with X representing that amount:

X = [3,570   x   (1 + 0.035)   /   1.7]   +   £0   = £2173.50
    Purchase   Commission   Conversion   Fee

Q1.3 – d: £859.29

The first spending will be with regard to the £380 he exchanged before he left. Since the banks deduct both the commission and the fee from the original £380 given to the bank, he will simply have spent £380.

Secondly, he withdrew $780 in cash from an ATM in the US. The actual cost of this withdrawal is:

$780 x 1.025 / 1.7 + £ 9 (3 withdrawals at £3 each) = £479.29
Total = £859.29.

Q1.4 – b: Bank B
You can obviously calculate the cost for each bank, which would lead you to the answer quickly enough. However, it is possible to exclude some options simply by looking at the data. Looking at the rates we can conclude the following:

▶ Bank B and Bank C have the same fee but Bank B has a lower level of commission and is therefore cheaper.

▶ Bank B has a cheaper commission rate and cheaper fee than Bank D. Therefore Bank B is cheaper than Bank D.

This now leaves us with Bank A and Bank B as possible candidates.
The cost for Bank A is 3,400 x 1.035 / 1.7 + 0 = 2,070
The cost for Bank B is 3,400 x 1.03 / 1.7 + 1 = 2,061

The answer is therefore: Bank B.

Q1.5 – b: £11.12
By paying cash he will benefit from a commission rate of 2% instead of 3.2%, i.e. a saving of 1.2% or $24. This is equivalent to 24 / 1.7 = £14.12. However, he will be required to pay a £4 fee instead of a £1 fee, i.e. £3 more. Hence the total saving in Pounds is 14.12 – 3 = £11.12.

Q1.6 – d: 2.34%
By reducing its fee to zero, the bank will lose £4, which it needs to make up through higher commission. If the commission increase rate is R then we need to solve the following equation: £4 = R x 2000 / 1.7, which gives R = 0.0034; i.e. an increase of 0.34% increase. The new rate should therefore be 2.34%.

QR 2 – Amusement Park

Q2.1 – b: decrease by 13.29%
The income for the two years is as follows (in thousands of pounds)
2004: 27x3.55 + 20x6.10 = 217.85
2005: 24x3.55 + 17x6.10 = 188.90
The ratio is 188.90 / 217.85 = 0.8671 i.e. a decrease in sales by 13.29%

$(1 - 0.8671 = 0.1329)$. Note that we are asked to measure the change from 2004 to 2005; this is measured as a percentage of the 2004 income.

Q2.2 – b: 13.34%
Total income for 2006 is calculated as follows (in thousands):
44x3.35 + 24x4.00 + 32 x 5.35 + 17x6.65 + 12x2.00 + 14.3x4.00 = 608.85
Total income from group tickets for 2006 is calculated as follows (in thousands): 12x2.00 + 14.3x4.00 = 81.2.
Proportion of group tickets sales = 81.2 / 608.85 = 13.34%

Q2.3 – a: 7.84%
You could calculate all the ratios between 2005 and 2004 ticket sales; or you can look at the numbers carefully and solve the problem through logic. Looking at the 2004 and 2005 ticket sales, we can see that the Children Low Season loss has been of 4,000 tickets out of 51,000 in 2004, which is under 10%. For all other categories, the loss has been over 10%. The Children Low Season category is the category which has experienced the smallest loss. The percentage is 4,000 / 51,000 = 7.84%

Q2.4 – a: 4.81%
2004 income for Adult High Season tickets = 20,000 x 6.10 = 122,000.
Ticket price required for 2008 = 122,000 / 17,504 = £6.97.
Increase required = 6.97 / 6.65 = 1.0481, i.e. an increase of 4.81%

Note that although the price increase is calculated to match the 2004 income, the actual increase itself is expressed as a percentage of the previous years' price and not the 2004 price.

Q2.5 – c: £3.55
The income for 2007 for individual children was:
46,000 x £3.35 + 21,000 x £4.00 = £238,100.
This now has to be distributed between 46,000 + 21,000 = 67,000 tickets.
The price is therefore 238,100 / 67,000 = £3.55.

Q2.6 – d: £72.00
The saving per adult in 2004 and 2005 is £5.10 – £4.05 = £1.05.
The saving per adult in 2006 and 2007 is £5.35 – £4.00 = £1.35.
Over four years, an adult will therefore save 2 x 1.05 + 2 x 1.35 = £4.80.
A group of 15 will therefore save 15 x £4.80 = £72.

Q2.7 – b: £2,760
The price per child was 70% of £2.00, i.e. £1.40.
The price per adult was 50% of £4.00, i.e. £2.00.
The total cost was therefore 900 x £1.40 + 750 x £2.00 = £2,760.

QR 3 – The Hunters and the Hunted

Q3.1 – a: 30,101 m^2
The area of the field is calculated as: (240 /1.0936) x (150/1.0936).

Q3.2 – a: 12,514 yd^2
(1 – 1/6 – 2/7 – 1/5) x (240 x 150) = 12,514 yd^2

Q3.3 – a: 2
If Hunter A killed 2 pheasants then, since this is 3 times fewer than Hunter B, then Hunter B has killed 6 pheasants, making a total of 8 pheasants killed.

Since they killed a total of 14 animals, this means they killed 6 rabbits between them.

We are told that Hunter A killed twice as many rabbits as Hunter B, therefore Hunter A killed 4 rabbits and Hunter B killed 2 rabbits.

Q3.4 – b: 901 rows
This is a simple interval problem. The trap to avoid is not to miss the final row. In 1 yard (i.e. 36 inches) we have 6 intervals of 6 inches each. In 150 yards, we therefore have 900 intervals of 6 inches each. The number of rows (i.e. lines delimiting the intervals) is therefore 901.

Q3.5 – b: 8min 34s
The full perimeter of the field measures (150 + 240) x 2 = 780 yd. This is equal to 780/1.0936 = 713.24m or 0.71324 km. At a speed of 5 km/h, he will run the distance in 0.71324 / 5 = 0.14266 hours i.e. x 60 = 8.559 minutes. This corresponds to 8 minutes 34 seconds.

Q3.6 – a: 705m
The length of the field is 240 / 1.0936 = 219.459m. The length of fence is therefore 2 metres less (1 metre on each side) i.e. 217.459m

The width of the field is 150 / 1.0936 = 137.162m. The length of fence is therefore 2 metres less (1 metre on each side) i.e. 135.162m.
The perimeter of the fence is therefore 2 x (217.459 + 135.162) i.e. 705.242m.

Q3.7 – e: 66 yd/min
At the time they meet, after 5 minutes, Hunter A has walked 5 x 60 = 300 yards. This means that Hunter B will have walked (240 + 150 + 240) – 300 = 330 yards during those same 5 minutes. His speed is therefore 330 / 5 = 66 yd/min.

QR 4 – Diamonds are Forever

Q4.1 – e: $21,125
A weight of 2.6g is equivalent to 2.6 / 0.2 = 13 carats.
A 13-carat diamond will cost 125 x 13^2 = $21,125.

Q4.2 – a: $7,000
Price of a 4-carat diamond = 125 x 4^2 = $2,000.
Price of a 7-carat diamond = 125 x 7^2 = $6,125.
Price of an 11-carat diamond = 3125 x 11^2 = $15,125.
Saving = 15,125 – (2,000 + 6,125) = $7,000.

Q4.3 – b: $12,500
Price of a 2.5-carat rough diamond = 125 x 2.5^2 = $781.25
Price of a 5-carat rough diamond = 125 x 5^2 = $3,125
Profit = 20 x 781.25 – 3125 = $12,500

Q4.4 – d: 7 carats
The new price would give the following equation:
$640 = (Price of 1 carat) x 4^2 i.e. price of 1 carat = $40.

This now gives us the equation 1960 = 40 x c^2, where c is the number of carats of the diamond. This gives c^2 = 1960 / 40 = 49, i.e. c = 7 carats.

Q4.5 – d: $1,652m
The question is asking about 2007 values, whilst we are only given 2008 values with % change. It is important to remember that these percentages will be based on the 2007 value. So, for example, if Oct–Dec 2008 polished exports have a value of $428m, and the % change is -62.1% then we have (Oct–Dec 2008 value) = (Oct–Dec 2007 value) x (1 – 0.621).

Therefore Oct–Dec 2007 value for polished imports = 428 / (1 – 0.621)
= 1129.29.

Similarly, Oct–Dec 2007 value for rough imports = 141 / (1 – 0.73)
= 522.22.

Total imports for Oct–Dec 2007 = 1129.29 + 522.22 = 1651.51.

Q4.6 – c: -3.88%
The value of polished imports across 2008 was 594 + 3,787 = $4,381m.
The value across 2007 was 594 / (1 – 0.428) + 3,787 / (1 + 0.076)
= $4,557.98m.

Ratio of 2008 over 2007 = 4381 / 4557.98 = 0.96117.
Change = 1 – 0.96116 = 0.03884, i.e. 3.88% decrease.

Q4.7 – b: $413m
The net export figure for the period Jan–Sep 2008 is calculated as:
(5,812 + 3,173) – (3,787 + 4,165) = 1,033.
An increase of 20% on the quarterly average will therefore give:
1,033 / 3 (there are 3 quarters in that period) x 1.20 = 413.20.

Q4.8 – c: $1,560m
This is simply calculated as the total Polished Exports over all quarters,
divided by 4. This gives: (428 + 5812) / 4 = $1,560.

QR 5 – Printing

Q5.1 – c: £12,504
Litho printing:
- Initial set-up cost = £1000
- Printing: 126 x 1600 = 201,600 pages at 4.5p each = £9,072

Cover
- 1600 at £1.40 each = £2,240
- Lamination (Gloss) = 1600 at £0.12 each = £192

Total= £12,504

Q5.2 – c: £360
The cost of Option A is: 3000 x (£1.00 + £0.20) = £3,600
The cost of Option B is: 3000 x (£1.00 x 1.2 + £0.12) = £3,960
Cost difference = 3,960 – 3,600 = £360

Q5.3 – c: 3681
If he made a profit a £34,500, then this means that the income he received from the bookshop is £9,672 + £34,500 = £44,172.

We know that the bookshop buys books at 75% of the RRP (£16), i.e. at £12 per book. Therefore the bookshop purchased 44,172 / 12 = 3,681

Q5.4 – b: £2,000
The quote was for 300 pages x 2000 books = 600,000 pages. This would have been quoted at 5p per page, i.e. £30,000. The actual number of pages printed was 400 pages x 2000 books = 800,000 pages, which should be priced at 4p per page, i.e. a total of £32,000. The difference on the printing of the pages is therefore £2,000. Note that the number of covers is the same (2000); therefore the difference is purely on the pages.

Q5.5 – c: 4p
The cost of printing the cover for 50 books (3 colours, laminated gloss is: 50 x (1.5 x 1.2 + 0.12) = £96. Since the total cost was £156, then this leaves £60 for the actual printing of the pages.

He wants to print 50 x 30 = 1500 pages. Therefore the cost per page is: 60 / 1500 = 0.04 i.e. 4p.

QR 6 – Fishy Business

Q6.1 – d: 6h15
The volume of the tank is 2,250 litres. At a rate of 6 litres per minute, it would take 375 minutes to fill, i.e. 6.25 hours i.e. 6 hours and 15 minutes.

Q6.2 – b: 90ml
The volume of water in the tank is 80% x 2250 = 1800 litres. We therefore need 1800 drops, i.e. 1800 x 0.05 = 90ml.

Q6.3 – c: 250cm^3
The volume of water displaced by the fish is 0.5 x 200 x 150 = 15000cm^3. Dividing by 60 fish gives an average volume of 15,000/60 = 250cm^3.

Q6.4 – a: 81
The tank must not go over the 80% mark, and we know that 15% of the total volume is taken by the gravel. Therefore the water will occupy 65% of the volume i.e. 65% x 2,250 =1462.50 litres.

We are allowed no more than 2.5cm of fish for 4.5 litres of water. There-fore the maximum length of fish allowed is 1462.50 / 4.5 x 2.5 = 812.50cm. This represents 81 fish of 10cm each. Note that we need to round down as having 82 fish into the tank would make us go over the limit allowed.

Q6.5 – c: 192
Each tile measures 12.5cm, which means that we can fit exactly 16 tiles in the 2m length of the tank; and exactly 12 in the 1.50m width. The total number of tiles is therefore 12 x 16 = 192.

Q6.6 – c: 88.5cm
The height of the tank is equal to its volume i.e. 2250 l (or 2,250,000cm^3 or 2.25m^3) divided by the two dimensions that we are given. This gives: 2,250,000 cm^3 / 200cm / 150cm = 75cm. Adding 18% gives 88.5cm.

Q6.7 – d: 6.4 kg
First we need to establish the volume of gravel needed for the tank. This will be given by the floor surface area of the tank multiplied by the desired height of gravel, i.e. (using cm) 150 x 200 x 3 = 90,000cm^3

Second we need to establish how much volume the 5kg bag can cover. This is equal to 10,000cm^2 (i.e. 1m^2) x 7 = 70,000cm^3.

Therefore we need 9/7th of a bag to cover the tank floor.
9 / 7 x 5kg = 6.4 kg.

Another way to solve is to say that the surface area of the tank is 3m^2 (2 x 1.5). Covering the surface with 3cm of gravel would use the same amount of gravel as covering 1m^2 with 9 cm of gravel. This would use 9/7th of a bag.

Q6.8 – c: £3,917
The cubic tank has a volume of 30cm x 30cm x 30cm =27,000cm^3. The enthusiast's tank has a volume of 2,250 litres, which is equivalent to 2,250,000cm^3. Its cost would therefore be 2250 / 27 x £47 = £3,917.

QR 7 – World News

Q7.1 – c: 68%
(98,700 + 130,000) / (98,700 + 130,000 + 110,000) = 0.675, i.e. 68%

Q7.2 – e: £87,828
The income is calculated as:
156,000 x (0.37x0.50 + 0.63x0.60) = £87,828.

Q7.3 – d: £124,495
The income from Europe comes from Newspaper B and 37% of Newspaper C. In Year 4, the income was 156,000 x 0.60 + 37% x 167,000 x 0.50 = £124,495.

Q7.4 – d: 719,000
Total sales in Year 6 will be:
133,000 x (1 – 0.50) + 176,000 x (1 + 1.33) + 156,000 x (1 + 5/9)
= 719,247.

Q7.5 – d: Year 11
We know that the retail price remains at Year 5 level i.e. 60p. We need to calculate N, the number of years that it will take to have 30p x 1.1^N>60p.

If you know about logarithms then you will find the answer quickly. However, logarithms are beyond the scope of the UKCAT, so if you are not familiar with them, don't worry; you can simply start with 30 on your calculator and keep adding 10% until you get a result which is above 60.

Year 4: 30 x 1.1 = 33
Year 5: 33 x 1.1 = 36.3
Year 6: 36.3 x 1.1 = 39.93
Year 7: 39.93 x 1.1 = 43.923
Year 8: 43.923 x 1.1 = 48.3153
Year 9: 48.3153 x 1.1 = 53.14683
Year 10: 53.13683 x 1.1 = 58.461513
Year 11: 58.461513 x 1.10 = 64.3076643 is over 60p.

By simply typing "x 1.1" continuously into the calculator, you should get to the result within 20 seconds.

Q7.6 – d: 41.4%
In Year 3, a total of 110,000+ 190,000+135,000 = 435,000 copies were sold. Out of this, 110,000 (Newspaper B) and 37% x 190,000 = 70,300 (Newspaper C) = 180,300 copies were sold in Europe.

This represents 180,300 / 435,000 = 41.4%

Q7.7 – b: £79,127
For Years 1 to 3, the price is the same regardless of the continent (55p).
For Years 4 and 5, the weighted price is 37% x 50p + 63% x 60p = 56.3p.

The total income was therefore:
(98700+100000+190000) x 0.55 + (167000+156000) x 0.563 = £395,634.
The average across the five years is therefore: 395,634 / 5 = £79,126.80.

QR 8 – D.I.Y.

Q8.1 – d: 481.72 ft^2
Instead of converting all dimensions into feet, it is quicker to make the calculation in metres and to convert the result into ft^2 using the conversion rate 1m^2 = (3.27)^2 ft^2, i.e. 10.6929 ft^2. The total surface area is equal to:
(3.2 + 1.2 + 1.8 + 3.3) x 3.6 + (3.5 x 3.1) = 45.05 m^2.
45.05 x 10.6929 = 481.72 ft^2.

Q8.2 – a: 1.86 cm^2
On a scale of 1:200, each dimension must be divided by 200.
The hall's surface on paper is therefore:
(3.20 + 1.20 + 1.80) / 200 x (1.20 / 200) = 0.000186 m^2 = 1.86 cm^2.

Q8.3 – e: 1.50 m
The combined surface area of the rectangle made up of the bedroom and the bathroom is (3.20+1.20) x (3.60–1.20) = 10.56 m^2. The surface of the bathroom alone is therefore: 10.56 – 8.76 = 1.80 m^2. The length of the longer wall is therefore equal to 1.80 / 1.20 (the length of the shorter wall) = 1.50m.

Q8.4 – d: 30.57 m^2
The total surface of the walls, ignoring any of the openings is calculated as the total length of the walls multiplied by the height of the walls (2.65m): (3.60 + 3.30) x 2 x 2.65 = 36.57 m^2.

The surface area occupied by the openings is:
(1.5 x 2) + (0.6 x 2) + (0.9 x 2) = 6 m^2.

The area occupied by the wallpaper is therefore 36.57 – 6 = 30.57 m^2.

Q8.5 – c: 32.4m
Top wall: 3.20 + 1.20 + 1.80 + 3.30 = 9.5m

Right wall: 3.6 + 3.1 = 6.7m

Bottom wall (L shaped): Horizontal walls add up to 9.5 m (i.e. same as top wall) + 3.1m for the lounge's left wall = 12.6m

Left wall: 3.6m

Total: 32.4m

The astute candidate will have spotted that in fact this is the same as twice the length of the top wall + twice the length of the right wall.

Q8.6 – b: £137.65
There are two ways to think about this problem, both of which lead to the same calculation.

Method 1 (using surface area)
The surface area occupied by the wooden floor should equal that of the room. The room's surface area is 3.5 x 3.1 = 10.85 m^2. One plank covers 1 x 0.10 = 0.10 m^2. Therefore we need 10.85 / 0.10 = 108.50 planks, i.e. we need to buy 5 packs (one not fully used). The cost is 5 x 27.53 = £137.65.

Method 2 (using length)
The lounge's length is 3.5m, therefore one row of planks will consist of 3.5 planks. The lounge's width is 3.1m. Since each plank has a width of 10cm, we can fit 10 planks in one metre and there in 3.1m we can fit 31 planks. The total number of planks required is therefore 3.5 x 31 = 108.5, i.e. 5 packs (one not fully used). The cost is 5 x 27.53 = £137.65.

QR 9 – Going for a Ride

Q9.1 – a: 17min 30s
The distance from E to C is 12 km. If this is done in 20 minutes then the average travelling speed is 36 km/h. The distance between E and H is 10.5 km. At a speed of 36 km/h, this can be travelled in 10.5/36 = 0.291666 hour. Multiplied by 60, this gives 17.5 minutes i.e. 17 minutes 30 seconds.

Q9.2 – c: 8.0 km/h
The journey totals 47+3+9+8+7.5+3+6.5 = 84 km. If the cyclist rides this distance in 10 hours 30 minutes (i.e. 10.5 hours) then his average speed is 84 / 10.5 = 8.0 km/h.

Q9.3 – d: Town F
Mr Smith has 2h25, but will only be driving for 2h25 – 49 minutes = 96 minutes return, or 48 minutes for one single journey i.e. 48/60th of an hour. Driving at 70 km/h he will travel 70 x (48/60) = 56 km. Starting from point G, this will correspond to Town F.

Q9.4 – c: Town E
The cyclist will have travelled 40/60 x 18 = 12 km in 40 minutes. Starting from Town C, this will take him to Town E (9km + 3km).

Q9.5 – d: 20 km/h
The distance between Town D and Town H is 47 + 3 + 7.5 = 57.5 km. At a speed of 18.4 km/h, this would take 57.5/18.4 = 3.125 hours, i.e. 3 hours and 7.5 minutes.

Reducing the journey by 15 minutes would make it last 3.125 - 0.25 = 2.875 hours. Riding 57.5 km in that amount of time gives an average speed of 57.5 / 2.875 = 20 km/h.

Note that if you ever had to guess, you could easily dismiss answer a, b and c. If he wants to reduce his journey time, he will need to travel faster than 18.4 km/h and therefore only answers 'd' and 'e' are suitable.

Q9.6 – c: 1h 28min
The distance to travel from C to G is equal to 65 km. The tube will therefore take 65/30 hours (i.e. 2.16666 hours, or 130 minutes) + (1 minute x 3 intermediary stops) = 133 minutes, i.e. 2 hours and 13 minutes.
The car will travel 47km at 100km/h and 18km at 50km/h and will therefore take 47/94 + 18/72 = 0.75 hours, i.e. 45 minutes.

The difference is therefore 88 minutes, or 1 hour 28 minutes.

Q9.7 – c: 36 times
Line FCH has a loop journey of 24.5 km. At 49 km/h, this will be achieved in 30 minutes.

The buses will therefore go through Town C twice every hour. Over the period 5am to 11pm (representing 18 hours), this represents 36 occasions.

QR 10 – Hot Chocolate

Q10.1 – d: 8.1g
A drink made of 18g of powder and 200ml of whole milk contains 9.6g of fat. 100g of powder contains 8.4g of fat, therefore 18g of powder contains 18/100 x 8.4 = 1.512g. The amount of fat in 200ml of whole milk is therefore 9.6 – 1.512 = 8.088g.

Q10.2 – a: 56 ml
The total fat content of 2.464g contains fat from the chocolate (18/100 x 8.4 = 1.512). Therefore the milk/water mix contains 2.464 – 1.512 = 0.952g of fat. Since we are told there is no fat in water, this can only come from the semi-skimmed milk. If 100ml of semi-skimmed milk contains 1.7g of fat, then to obtain 0.952g, we need a volume of 0.952 x 100 / 1.7 = 56ml.

Q10.3 – c: 7.0 pints
The box contains 360g of chocolate (i.e. 20 x 18g).
He therefore needs 20 x 200ml = 4,000ml of milk which is equivalent to 4000/570 = 7.0 pints.

Q10.4 – c: 2 drinks
One chocolate drink made from water will have the same amount of calories as the 18g of chocolate powder used to make it, i.e. 372 x 18 / 100 = 66.96 kCal. The three water-based drinks together will therefore account for 3 x 66.96 = 200.88 kCal.

This leaves an allowance of 800 – 200.88 = 599.12 kCal for all other whole-milk-based drinks. We know from the table that each contains 200 kCal and therefore he is just short of being able to make 3 drinks.

Since 3 drinks will just about push him over the limit, the answer is 2 drinks.

Q10.5 – c: 164g
The box contains 360g of chocolate; therefore, at a rate of 18g per drink, the client can make 20 drinks out of the whole box. For these 20 drinks he will require 20 x 200ml of milk, i.e. 4 litres.

The protein included in the whole box (360g) of chocolate amounts to 360/100 x 8.9g = 32.04g. The protein included in the 4 litres of semi-skimmed milk amounts to 40 x 3.3g = 132g.

The total amount of protein is therefore 164.04g.

Q10.6 – c: 9 kCal
This can be calculated using either of the two columns.
Column 1: (372 – 4x8.9 – 4x65.2) / 8.4 = 9
Column 2: (200 – 4x8.0 – 4x20.4) / 9.6 = 9

QR 11 – Time Traveller

Q11.1 – e: 6h 20min
The time in Los Angeles is 3 hours behind the time in New York. Therefore if a flight leaving New York at 11:30 (New York time) arrives at 14:50 (Los Angeles time), when the plane arrives in Los Angeles it will be 17:50 in New York (i.e. 3 hours more).

Therefore, when expressed in New York time, the flight times are 11:30 to 17:50 i.e. a duration of 6 hours and 20 minutes.

Q11.2 – c: 13h 35min
There are two ways of calculating the result, one being far longer than the other.

The long way
Travel time from London to Paris = 10:15 – 7:50 = 2:25 – 1 hour difference = 1 hour 25 minutes.
Arrival at 10:15 in Paris means departure at 11:15 from Paris, hence waiting time of 1 hour.

Travel time from Paris to LA: 13:25 – 11:15 = 2:10 + time difference of 9 hours = 11 hours 10 minutes.

Total time travelled = 1:25 + 1:00 + 11:10 = 13 hours 35 minutes.

The short way
Essentially, since we are asked to calculate the total travelling time, it does not matter what happens between departure and arrival. Leaving at 7:50 from London makes him arrive in Paris at 10:15, where he can transfer to the 11:15 to LA, which arrives at 13:25.

The travelling time is therefore 13h 25min – 7h 50min = 5h 35min plus the time difference between London and Los Angeles (8 hours) = 13h 35min.

Q11.3 – d: 5,840km
The travel time between Paris and New York is 2 hours (difference between departure and arrival time) + 6 hours' time difference = 8 hours. Since the average speed is 730 km/h, the distance is 8 x 730 = 5,840km.

Q11.4 – e: 4h 15min
For this question, there is no need to deal with time differences at all, since the initial and final destinations are the same for both.

Jack flies via Paris using the 9:25 from London to Paris. He arrives in Paris at 11:50 and can then catch the 13:00 to LA, which arrives at 15:10.

John flies via New York using the 9:10 from London to NY. He arrives at 12:10 in NY, where he can then catch the 15:50 from NY to LA, which arrives at 19:10.

John therefore left 15 minutes earlier than Jack but arrived 4 hours later. He will therefore have travelled 4 hours 15 minutes more than Jack.

Q11.5 – d: 17:40
The last flight from NY to LA leaves at 20:10 therefore the new Paris to NY flight should arrive in NY at 19:40 (30 minutes before). Since the difference in time between the departure and arrival time is always 2 hours, this means that the plane should leave Paris at 17:40 local time.

Q11.6 – d: 68,474
All flights from Paris to Los Angeles take 11 hours and 10 minutes. Four daily flights represent 44 hours and 40 minutes of flight.

The fuel consumed is therefore: (44+40/60) x 730 x 2.1 = 68,474 litres.

QR 12 – Conferencing & Banqueting

Q12.1 – d: £400
Although the number of participants is 7, the contract has a minimum of 8 participants required. Therefore the cost is £50 x 8 = £400.

Q12.2 – d: £799
The cost of each of the DDR items on a room basis is as follows:

Room: £250
Projector: £189
Flipchart: £15
30 coffee breaks (3 breaks x 10): 30 x £2.50 = £75
Orange juice (2 jugs) = 2 x £10 = £20
10 sit-down lunches: 10 x £20 = £200
Water: 10 bottles: 10 x £5 = £50
Total = £799

Q12.3 – e: 16
There are two ways of resolving this question:

Method 1 – Write an equation
The crossover point "P" where the DDR cost is equal to the RB cost is calculated as follows: 45 P = £250 + £15 + (2.50 x 3 + 20) x P.
i.e. 17.5 P = £265, hence P = 15.14.

At P = 15, the DDR cost is cheaper than the RB cost.
At P = 16, the DDR cost is greater than the RB cost.

Note: once you have identified which costs are fixed and which costs depend on the number of participants, you can also find the solution using trial and error, based on the options on offer.

Method 2 – Average cost calculation
Under a DDR contract, the cost per person is £45. Therefore we must find the number of participants which gives a cost of £45 under the RB contract.

If we take off the cost of food and drink (£20 + 3 x £2.50 = £27.50 per person), we are left with an average cost of £45 - £27.50 = £17.50 to pay the room and the projector.

The total cost for the room and the flipchart is £250 + £15 = £265. Therefore the limit is calculated as follows: 265 / 17.50 = 15.14.

Q12.4 – c: £44.04
The new rate is 45 / 1.175 x 1.15 = £44.04.

Q12.5 – d: £37.84
The average cost per person will be the £30 cost charged by the caterer + the cost of the room (including surcharge) split between 50 people, i.e. (30 + 350 x 1.12) / 50 = £37.84.

QR 13 – Milking It

Q13.1 – d: 5.089 kg
The daily production of milk is 15 x 8.75 = 131.25 litres, which weighs 131.25 x 1.034 = 135.7125 kg. 15% of this is cream, of which only 25% is butter. The weight of the butter is therefore 135.7125 x 0.15 x 0.25, i.e. 5.089 kg.

Q13.2 – c: 1,343.55
In April (i.e. 30 days), the weight of milk produced would have been: 30 x 15 x 8.75 x 1.034 = 4,071.375 kg. At £0.33 per kilogram, this would cost £1,343.55.

Q13.3 – c: 1.027 kg
If the volume of water added is 25% of the volume of raw milk, then in 1 litre of the new mix there are 800ml of milk and 200ml of water. This weighs: 0.8 x 1.034 + 0.2= 1.0272kg

Q13.4 – c: 2,920.5 kg
On average, a cow will consume 19,800 / 160 / 15 = 8.25 kg per day during winter. He now has to feed 3 additional cows for 118 days, hence the hay required for that period will be 3 x 118 x 8.25 = 2,920.5 kg.

QR 14 – A Colourful Life

Q14.1 – b: 200ml
The volume of yellow paint contained in 2 litres of Amazon is 10% of 2 litres, i.e. 200ml.

Q14.2 – c: 22%
The total volume of paint obtained is 500ml.

The amount of red paint included in 100ml of Crimson is 70% of 100ml i.e. 70ml. The amount of red paint included in 400ml of Amazon is 10% of 400ml, i.e. 40ml.

In total, there is therefore 70 + 40 = 110ml of red paint in a total volume of 500ml. This is equivalent to 22%.

Q14.3 – e: 1.212 litres
A pot of 1 litre of Violet will contain:
- 400 ml of red
- 400 ml of blue
- 200 ml of yellow

Since we are only adding yellow paint to it, the volume of red and blue paints will not change.

Therefore, once we have obtained the Chocolate colour, it will be made up of 400ml of red, 400ml of blue and an unknown quantity of yellow.

We know that Chocolate contains 33% of both red and blue paint; therefore once the colour has been created, the 400ml of red will represent 33% of the final volume. The final volume is therefore 400 / 0.33 = 1,212ml or 1.212 litres.

Q14.4 – c: 43.6%
The fact that the paints are mixed in equal quantities makes it easier to calculate.
If we take a sample of 100ml of each of the paints then the paint resulting from the mix will contain the following volume of blue paint:
33 + 80 + 45 + 40 + 20 = 218ml out of a total volume of 500ml.
The percentage is therefore 218 / 500 = 0.436 i.e. 43.6%.

QR 15 – Advertising Rates

Q15.1 – d: £720
The cost of a colour advert spanning two columns, with a height of 8cm is:
£75 x 8 x 1.2 = £720.

Q15.2 – c: £1,000
There are two options available:
- Option 1: Purchase 7 cm across 4 columns, which would cost £150 x 7 = £1,050.
- Option 2: Pay for a quarter page (7cm is one quarter of the total 28cm available). The cost would be £1,000. This is the cheapest option.

Q15.3 – b: £1,800
Scenario 1: The income generated is: 4 columns x 28cm x £50 = £5,600.
Scenario 2: The income generated is £3,800.
The loss would therefore be £1,800.

Q15.4 – e: £2,325
Watch out for the minimum charge of 3 cm which will apply to the single column advert of 2 cm. The income gained from the adverts will be:
(1000 x 1.2) + (75 x 5) + 3 x (50 x 4) + (50 x 3) (min charge) = £2,325.

Q15.5 – e: £20,160
The maximum income will be generated by selling all adverts on a single column basis, with all adverts having a height of 1 cm and being charged at a minimum rate of 3 cm, in full colour.

This is equivalent to 28 adverts per column, i.e. 112 adverts per page at a maximum cost of 3 x £50 x 1.2 = £180 each. The maximum income is therefore 112 x 180 = £20,160.

QR 16 – A matter of Time

Q16.1 – b: 6 minutes
The additional journey time is 5 minutes for the first part of the journey (20 – 15) plus 1 minute for the second part of the journey (14 – 13). The final two parts took the same amount of time in both years.

Q16.2 – d: 76 km/h
The total distance was 12 + 18 + 34 = 64 miles.
This was travelled in 13 + 25 + 43 = 81 minutes (or 81/60 hours).
The average speed was therefore: 64 x 1.6093 / 81 x 60 = 76 km/h.

Q16.3 – d: 10.20%
The journey time in 1987 on the Southend to Fenchurch Street line was 49 minutes. In 2008, it was 54 minutes. This represents an increase of 54 / 49 = 1.102, i.e. 10.2%

Q16.4 – b: 86.9 km/h
In 1987, the total journey time was 5 minutes less than in 2008. We are told that this time must be recovered on the Faversham to Chatham portion of the route and therefore this part of the journey (18 miles) will need to be done in 20 minutes instead of 25 minutes. 18 miles in 20 minutes is equivalent to 54 miles in an hour. Converting to kilometres (x 1.6093) gives a speed of 86.9 km/h.

Q16.5 – a: 50 miles
The number of miles on the Canterbury to Victoria Line is 64. Therefore the cost on a pound per mile basis is calculated as 15.90/64 = £0.2484375.

A ticket on the Lewes to Victoria line costs £12.40. Since the cost on a pound per mile basis is the same on both lines, the number of miles on the Lewes to Victoria line is 12.40 / 0.2484375 = 49.91 miles (rounded up to 50 miles).

QR 17 – Within Shopping Distance

Q17.1 – d: 650
The number of shops is obtained by looking at the white bars and the left axis for each of the distances. It is equal to: 200 + 100 + 50 + 100 + 50 + 100 + 50 = 650 shops.

Q17.2 – e: £150m
We are asked for the total turnover (i.e. average turnover x number of shops) for shops within a 5-mile radius so both the 0-1 and the 1-5 categories need to be included. Expressed in thousands of pounds:
Total turnover for 0-1-mile radius = 600 x 200 = 120,000.
Total turnover for 1-5-mile radius = 300 x 100 = 30,000.
Total = 120,000 + 30,000 = 150,000. This is in thousands of pounds, hence the answer is £150m.

Q17.3 – a: 0-1
This is the type of question where it pays to look at the graph carefully. The section 0-1 has both the highest average turnover and the highest number of shops so it is the obvious answer.

Q17.4 – e: 70.6%
There is no substitute for doing all calculations here. To accelerate the process, you can, however, place together all data which have a common element:

Total turnover (in thousands)
= 200x600 + 100x(300+400+200) + 50x(600+200+100) = 255,000.

Turnover for shops within a 10-mile radius (i.e. the first three categories) in thousands) = 200x600 + 100x300 + 600x50 = 180,000.

Percentage = 180,000 / 255,000 = 70.6%

Q17.5 – a: £5,500
First, we are told that all shops have a turnover over £100,000. So all of them will pay the 0.5% tax on the full £100,000 i.e. £500.

On average, the shops have a turnover of 600,000. So the portion above 100,000 will average 600,000 – 100,000 = 500,000 across all shops. A tax of 1% will correspond to an amount of £5,000.

In total the average tax is therefore £5,500 per shop.

Q17.6 – c: 595
The total number of shops within 10 miles is 200+100+50 = 350.
The total number of shops beyond 10 miles is 100+50+100+50 = 300.
Total number of shops after the change = 0.8x350 + 1.05x300 = 595.

Q17.7 – e: Can't tell
Because the zones are concentric around the reference point, two shops that are within the 10-15 zone could actually be up to 30 miles apart. The best we can conclude is that the pensioner will never be able to visit shops in zone 0-1, 20-25 and 25-30, but we can't conclude on how many shops he will actually have access to during the other zones.

QR 18 – Shaken, not Stirred

Q18.1 – d: 250ml
The volume of vodka required is: 50x2 + 25x5 + 1x25 = 250ml

Q18.2 – b: 35.25ml
Alcohol volume = 25x40% + 25x15% + 50x43% = 35.25ml

Q18.3 – d: 64
The 8 Tequila Sunrise cocktails will have used 800ml of orange juice, leaving 3.2 litres for the Screwdriver cocktails (which is the only other cocktail that can be made with orange juice in this bar). This can make 3,200/50 = 64 Screwdriver cocktails.

Q18.4 – c: Velocity
As for all questions which look as if many calculations are required, you should try to identify ways of cutting down on the work required. A quick scan of the table will identify that:
- All five options contain vermouth
- Most alcohols have an alcohol content of around 40% whereas vermouth only contains 15%. Therefore those containing proportionately more vermouth would contain less alcohol.
- Most of the cocktails in the list of options have a volume 75ml.

If you had to hazard a guess, Velocity would be a good candidate for the cocktail with the least volume of alcohol.
Check:
- Martini: 25x15%+ 50x43%= 25.25ml
- Vodkatini: 50x45% + 25x15% = 26.25ml
- *Velocity: 50x15% + 25x43% = 18.25ml*
- Orange Bloom: 25x40% + 25x15% + 50x43%= 35.25ml
- Journalist: 5x40% + 25x15% + 50x43% = 27.25ml

Q18.5 – d: +22.4%
Volume of alcohol in Balalaika: 25x40% + 25x45% = 21.25ml
Volume of alcohol in XYZ = 25x40% + 40x40% = 26ml
Increase = 26 / 21.25 = 1.224 i.e. 22.4% increase

Q18.6 – b: 1.3 litres
We need to make 3 litres of Velocity and 1.5 litres of Long Island.

A Velocity cocktail has a volume of 75ml (50+25) and a Long Island cocktail has a volume of 125ml. Therefore we need to make the equivalent of 3000/75 = 40 Velocity cocktails and 1500/125 = 12 Long Island cocktails.

This gives us a Gin volume of 40x25 + 12x25 = 1300ml, or 1.3 litres.

QR 19 – Entente Cordiale

Q19.1 – d: 5h 41min
The UK leg of the journey is 130km. The French leg of the journey is 300km. The journey time is therefore: 130/110 + 300/120 + 2hours (ferry) = 5.681818 hours i.e. 5 hours and 41 minutes.

Q19.2 – b: 20km
The fuel tank has a capacity of 45 litres, which will enable the courier to drive a distance of 45 x 10 = 450km.
The total distance from London to Paris is 430km. Therefore he will be able to get to Paris safely but will run out of petrol 20km thereafter.

Q19.3 – b: £65.54
The courier starts with a tank containing 20 litres of fuel. By the time he reaches the first petrol station, he will have travelled 80km and therefore used 80/10 = 8 litres, leaving 12 litres in the tank. He therefore needs a top up of 45-12 = 33 litres. The cost is 33 x 89p = £29.37.

By the time he reaches the second petrol station, he will have travelled 150km, using 15 litres. Refuelling will cost 15 x 1.25 / 1.20 = £15.62.

He then needs to travel 180km and therefore use 18 litres of fuel to get to the final petrol station, where refuelling costs 18 x 1.37 / 1.20 = £20.55. The total spend equals £29.37 + £15.62 + £20.55 = £65.54.

Q19.4 – b: €23.13
The spend for Car A is calculated as follows:
(20/15) x 0.95 + (180/15) x 0.87 + (150/15) x (0.99x1.20) = €23.59.
The spend for Car B is calculated as follows:
(20/10) x 1.76 + (180/10) x 1.47 + (150/10) x (0.93x1.20) = €46.72.
The difference is €23.13.

Q19.5 – b: 23 litres
There are only 3 possibilities for refuelling on the way:

Between London and Dover: this would only be for 8 litres and would cost £7.12, well below the €28.75 that he paid.

At the petrol station after Calais: this would be for 23 litres, calculated as (80+50+100)/10. It would cost 23 x €1.25 = €28.75 (the answer we are looking for).

At the petrol station before Paris, this would be for 41 litres and would cost 41 x €1.37 = €56.17.

Another way to get to the answer is to spot that, roughly speaking a litre of unleaded will cost between €1 and €1.4. A cost of €28.75 would therefore mean a refuelling of between 20 and 29 litres. This can only happen at the middle petrol station. At that petrol station the refuelling would need to be for 23 litres in view of the distance driven to get there and the consumption of 1 litre per 10km.

QR 20 – Parking

Q20.1 – d: 80p.
A 37-minute stay will be charged as 40 minutes and will therefore will cost 4 x 20p = 80p

Q20.2 – e: £1.30
According to the system set out in Note 3, the first period of 5 minutes (5:55pm – 6:00pm) will be charged at 30p and the second part of the stay (6:00pm – 6:15pm) will be charged at the standard £1. Hence the total is £1.30.

Q20.3 – e: £83.10
The Monday – Friday 9am – 6pm stays will each cost:
- 9am to 1pm: 4 hours x 6 periods x 20p = £4.80
- 1pm to 6pm: 5 hours x 6 periods x 30p = £9.00
Total cost= £13.80 per day.

The Saturday and Sunday 9am - 6pm stays will each cost: 9 hours x 3 periods x 15p = £4.05 per day. We also need to account for 6 overnight stays i.e. £6 in total. Total cost = 5 days x £13.80 + 2 days x £4.05 + £6 overnight = £83.10.

Q20.4 – d: £20
The week-day cost from 9am to 6pm is £13.80 (see previous question for calculation). However, he can use the ticket from 8:30am to 9:00am, which would normally be charged at the standard £1 fee. The total for the day is therefore £14.80. Over 5 days, this costs 5 x 14.80 = £74, hence a saving of £20.

Q20.5 – e: 50p
Note 3 tells us that he will be charged a full 20p for the first 2 minutes and a full 30p for the next 2 minutes (since both are in a different zones and therefore calculated separately with their own minimum charge).

Q20.6 – e: Saturday 1:40pm
Cost of Friday 5pm to 6pm = 6 x 30p = £1.80
Cost of overnight stay (Friday – Saturday) = £1. Cumulative total: £2.80
This leaves £2.10 to spend on the Saturday daytime. The cost of 15p per period, he can spend 2.10/0.15 = 14 periods of 20 minutes, i.e. 4 hours and 40 minutes in total. He must therefore have left the car park by Saturday 1:40pm.

ABSTRACT REASONING

TIPS & TECHNIQUES

+

130
PRACTICE QUESTIONS & ANSWERS

6 Abstract Reasoning
Format, Purpose & Key Techniques

FORMAT

The abstract reasoning part of the UKCAT contains 13 exercises. In each exercise, you will be given two sets of abstract shapes, named Set A and Set B.

All shapes within Set A are linked in one way; all shapes within Set B are linked in another way. Your first task is to determine the nature of the relationships between all shapes within each set. Once you have done so, you are given 5 test shapes and are asked to determine whether they belong to Set A, Set B or neither set.

EXAMPLE

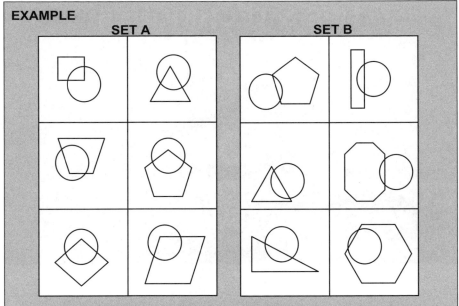

SET A   SET B

In this example, you can clearly see that every single shape within each set contains 2 objects: a circle and another object, and that both overlap. However, in Set A the circle crosses the other object on 2 separate edges;

whereas in Set B the circle crosses the other object on the same edge.

It is worth noting that, although the relationship that unites all shapes in Set A is different to the relationship that unites all shapes in Set B, there is a similarity, i.e. both relationships refer to the manner in which the objects intersect. In the exam, this is a useful feature which will help you out for some of the more difficult exercises.

Once you have determined the relationships within each set, you can then proceed to the test shapes to decide which set they belong to, if any. For example:

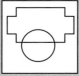

Test shape 1
This test shape belongs to Set B because the circle crosses the shape on one edge only.

Test Shape 2
This shape belongs to neither set because the circle crosses the triangle on 3 different edges.

In some cases, the shapes will contain objects or features which are "distractors", i.e. they do not play any particular role and are simply there to confuse you. You will therefore need to recognise quickly which objects matter and which do not.

The time given at the exam to do all 13 exercises (corresponding to 65 test shapes) is 16 minutes. This includes 1 minute to read the instructions and 15 minutes to carry out the test.

PURPOSE

The test is designed to assess your ability to develop ideas, test them and change your approach if necessary. This is a skill that you will need to use and demonstrate throughout your medical career. For example:

- As a doctor you will often be presented with a set of symptoms and/or results which you will need to use to forge an opinion about possible diagnoses. An ability to recognise patterns in the data available to you will help you identify those diagnoses.

- Once you have determined a number of possible diagnoses (so-called "differential diagnoses"), you will need to test whether they are viable before discounting them or accepting them.

- Much of the data will come from a medical history that you will have taken from a patient and from the results of tests that you will have ordered. Some of the information will be relevant, but some of it won't. Your strength as a doctor will lie in your ability to sieve through the information to use the relevant data and discard the irrelevant information.

- If you are involved in research, you may need to identify patterns in the data provided so that you can establish links between two or more parameters.

KEY TECHNIQUES

In the exam, you will only have 15 minutes to allocate 65 shapes (13 exercises, 5 shapes in each) to the relevant set. This gives you an average of 13 seconds per shape, which is very little. It is therefore crucial that you have at your disposal a number of techniques that you can use to work out the correct relationships and that you are fully aware of the possible combinations that can come up in the exam; this will help you discard the wrong relationships early on, and will assist you in recognising the more viable relationships at the earliest opportunity.

In this section, we have set out a number of techniques that you will need to practise when you do the abstract reasoning practice exercises and will help you save time at the exam:

Consider then validate or reject the simple/obvious relationships
Before you start making life complicated for yourself, make sure that you have considered the obvious. The possibilities are endless but here are some of the key relationships that you cannot afford to miss:

Type and size of the objects
- Are all objects within the shapes of the same type or different types?
- Are some objects of the same size or are they all different sizes?
- Is there one type of object which stands out in all shapes and could be a key object?
- Is there an object which consistently appears in each shape but with different colours and could be a key object?

Number of objects
- Is the number of objects the same in all shapes?
- Is the number of objects of one type the same in all shapes?
- Is there a relative relationship between two different types of objects (e.g. number of white objects = number of black objects + 1)?
- Is the number of objects of one type linked to a feature of another object (e.g. is the number of circles within each shape equal to the number of sides of another object within the shape)?
- If there are arrows, have you considered relationships which are linked not just to the number of arrows but also the number of arrowheads (some arrows may be double-ended)?

Number of sides
- Do all the objects have the same number of sides?
- Do all the objects have an odd or even number of sides?
- Do all the objects have a number of sides which is a multiple of 2, 3 or another number?
- Do the above relationships apply when taking all the shapes together as opposed to each object individually (e.g. is the sum of the number of sides for all objects within one shape the same)?
- Is the number of sides of one object linked to another object (e.g. is the number of sides of Object 1 equal to the number of sides of Object 2 + 1)?

Symmetries
- Are some objects a symmetrical image of other objects, either through line symmetry (i.e. mirror image) or rotational symmetry?

Number and type of angles
- Are all the angles under/over 90 or 180 degrees?
- Are there a fixed number of right angles?

87

- Does the number of right angles match the number of other objects within the shape?

Intersections
- Is the number of intersections the same in all shapes within the set?
- Do only certain types of objects intersect (e.g. those in a given colour, or those with a given number of edges)?
- Do the objects only intersect in a certain way (e.g. intersections are on straight edges but not on curved edges)?
- Do the objects which result from the intersection (i.e. the overlapping area) form a specific pattern which is the same across all shapes (e.g. they all have four sides, or are they coloured in the same way – striped, black, white)?

Colour of the objects
- Does the colour of the objects influence the counting of some of the key features (e.g. if you add the number of edges of the white shapes to double the number of edges of black shapes, do you get the same number)?
- Are some types of objects always of one particular colour (e.g. are all objects with four sides coloured in black)?

Position and direction of the objects
- Are some specific objects always in the same place? For example, is there always a triangle in the top right corner? If there is a circle in the shape, is it always in the centre of the shape or in a corner?
- Do some objects always point in the same direction? For example, are the triangles always pointing upwards? If an arrow is present, is it always pointing in the same direction?
- Is there always one type of object placed the same way relative to another object (i.e. is there always a square to the right of a triangle? Or are the objects arranged in the same clockwise manner in each of the shapes)?
- Are some objects inside others?
- Is one object overlapping another object in the same way in every shape? (e.g. is the black object always overlapping a white object? If yes, is it always the black or white object which is on top? Or it is always the object with the least number of sides which is on top?)
- If the shapes contain a lot of arrows, are they all pointing in the same direction? Or perhaps they are pointing in all directions but one?

Consider relationships of dependence between objects

There are sets of shapes in which the status of one object will depend on another object, which acts as a key. For example:

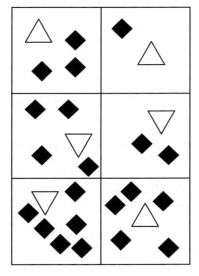

In this set of shapes, there is always one white triangle and a number of black diamonds. It is therefore clearly a requirement that, in order to belong to this set, all shapes should have one and only one white triangle of this type, and that any diamonds present in the shape should be black and of the standard size of those present in the shape here.

However, you may have spotted too that some triangles are pointing upwards and others downwards. A quick count of the black shapes will reveal that, when the triangle points upwards, the number of diamonds is odd, whilst when the triangle points downwards the number of diamonds is even.

Another example:

In this set, there are several relationships, all of which are linked to the arrow.

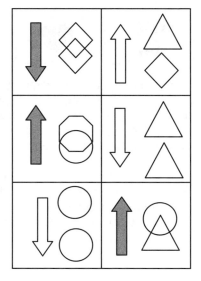

- There is always one arrow next to two objects which feature one above the other and which are always white.

- If the arrow points upwards then the two objects are different, whilst if the arrow points downwards then the objects are identical

- If the arrow is white then the objects do not overlap, whilst if the arrow is grey then the two objects overlap.

In this last example, the fact that the same arrow presents in each shape under different guises should be a clue that it may be a key shape that dictates a number of relationships.

Watch out for distractors

Distractors are objects which are simply sitting there and have no particular relationship with the others, or are features which you may be paying attention to but in fact have no bearing on the relationship between the objects present in each shape.

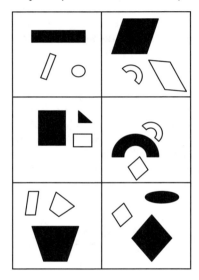

For example, in this set, the relationship is that:

- There is always one black object and one white object that are of the same type (two rectangles, two diamonds, etc.), with the white replica being smaller in size.

- There is always another object present, but the type of the object, its colour, its size and position do not matter (i.e. no pattern can be established). Note that it is important that there is an additional object, but none of its features matter.

The good news is that distractors are not very common, and, when they are present, they tend to be fairly simple to spot. The main problem is that they will waste your valuable time and, in some cases, you will always be wondering whether there is something that you have missed. The most common distractors are as follows:

- The colours of the objects within the shape do not matter.
- The shapes of the objects do not matter.
- There are additional objects floating around which simply fill the space but are not part of any relationship.

Use both sets together to work out the relationships
In the exam, the two sets have exclusive relationships, i.e. the relationship common to all shapes within Set A is different to the relationship common to all shapes within Set B. However, the two relationships are usually related in a mirrored fashion. For example, you could have the following relationships:

Example 1
Set A: All objects within the shape have an odd number of edges. All those with curved edges are black; the others are white.
Set B: All objects within the shape have an even number of edges. All those with curved edges are white; the others are black.

Example 2
Set A: The shapes all contain triangles and circles. The number of circles is equal to the number of isosceles triangles within the shape. Colour is irrelevant.
Set B: The shapes all contain triangles and circles. The number of circles is equal to the number of triangles with a right angle.

Example 3
Set A: There are 7 objects within each shape. All objects which overlap another are white; the others are black.
Set B: There are 8 objects within each shape. All objects which overlap another are black. The others are white.

Example 4
Set A: If the arrow points upwards, then all circles are black. A striped triangle means that the circles are on the right. A striped arrow means that the circles are on the left.
Set B: If the arrow points downwards, then all triangles are white. A striped arrow means that the circles are on the right.

Looking at both sets together can enable you to find relationships more easily because you know that, if you identify a relationship in one set, you are likely to have a similar type of relationship in the other set (albeit using opposite parameters). It may also enable you to spot relationships that you would not necessarily have spotted by looking at one set only.

If you struggle, take a step back and look at the whole picture
There are times when your brain might simply not be looking in the right place, or where you will obsessively attempt to find relationships where there aren't any, which could cause frustration.

If you are struggling to find relationships which link all the shapes within one set, step back from the page/screen and look at it from a slight distance. You may see patterns that did not come to mind before such as a dominant colour or a similarity between some shapes.

Use your time appropriately
In the exam, you have 15 minutes to deal with 65 test shapes corresponding to 13 exercises (5 shapes per exercise). This gives you 1 minute and 9 seconds per exercise, or just under 14 seconds per shape. In reality the bulk of the work is in determining the relationships within each set; once you have done that, determining whether each of the 5 test shapes fits within Set A, Set B or neither should be fairly quick.

It would therefore be wise to spend 45 seconds or so to determine how the shapes are linked within each set, and then to spend the remaining 25 seconds allocating the test shapes to the correct set (this makes it 5 seconds per test shape).

Practise, practise, practise
Although there is no knowledge to be acquired or remembered to do well in the abstract reasoning test, it is important that you become used to identifying the relationships quickly so that you can obtain a high score. In the next section you will find 26 exercises (130 test shapes) which will give you an opportunity to do so.

7 Abstract Reasoning Practice Questions

This section contains 26 exercises, each of which contains 5 test shapes, hence a total of 130 questions. This is equivalent to two full exams. These questions are designed to help you develop an awareness of the different techniques and tips mentioned in the previous section and to familiarise you with the different approaches that actual exam questions can take.

If you have already practised for abstract reasoning exercises through other means, you may wish to practise these questions in real time, in which case you should aim to complete each exercise (i.e. all 5 test shapes) in less than 1 minute 10 seconds. Alternatively, you may choose to replicate exam conditions and split this section into two lots of 13 questions, which you aim to complete in under 15 minutes each.

The answers to all questions, together with explanations, can be found from page 120 onwards.

Once you have practised on all 130 test shapes questions, you should be ready to confront the mock exam which features at the back of this book and replicates the actual exam's format (i.e. 13 exercises, 5test shapes each). You may want to wait until you have practised all sections in this book before going ahead with the mock exam.

AR 1 Practice	Practice Exercise 1

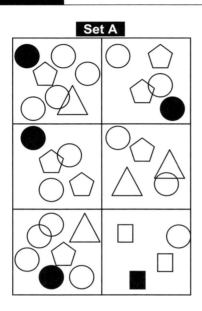

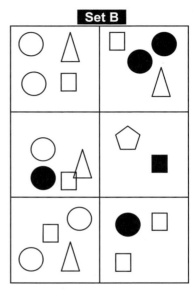

To which of the two sets above do the following shapes belong?

Shape 1.1	Shape 1.2	Shape 1.3	Shape 1.4	Shape 1.5

☐ Set A   ☐ Set A   ☐ Set A   ☐ Set A   ☐ Set A

☐ Set B   ☐ Set B   ☐ Set B   ☐ Set B   ☐ Set B

☐ Neither   ☐ Neither   ☐ Neither   ☐ Neither   ☐ Neither

AR 2
Practice

Practice Exercise 2

Set A

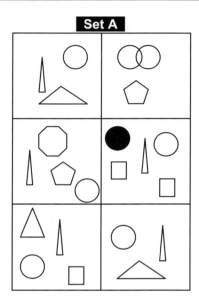

Set B

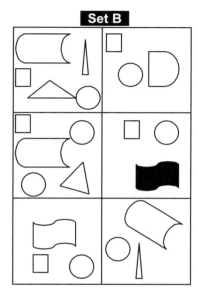

To which of the two sets above do the following shapes belong?

Shape 2.1	Shape 2.2	Shape 2.3	Shape 2.4	Shape 2.5

☐ Set A ☐ Set A ☐ Set A ☐ Set A ☐ Set A

☐ Set B ☐ Set B ☐ Set B ☐ Set B ☐ Set B

☐ Neither ☐ Neither ☐ Neither ☐ Neither ☐ Neither

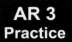

AR 3
Practice

Practice Exercise 3

Set A

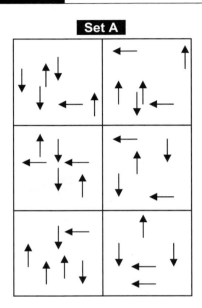

Set B

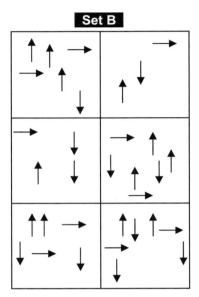

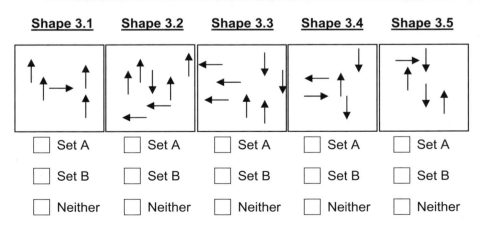

To which of the two sets above do the following shapes belong?

| Shape 3.1 | Shape 3.2 | Shape 3.3 | Shape 3.4 | Shape 3.5 |

☐ Set A   ☐ Set A   ☐ Set A   ☐ Set A   ☐ Set A

☐ Set B   ☐ Set B   ☐ Set B   ☐ Set B   ☐ Set B

☐ Neither ☐ Neither ☐ Neither ☐ Neither ☐ Neither

AR 4 Practice	**Practice Exercise 4**

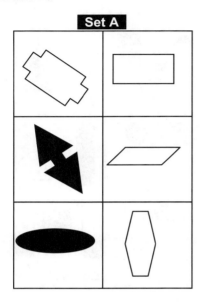

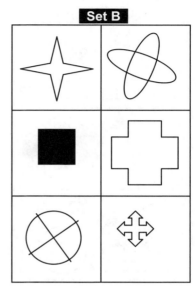

To which of the two sets above do the following shapes belong?

Shape 4.1	Shape 4.2	Shape 4.3	Shape 4.4	Shape 4.5

☐ Set A	☐ Set A	☐ Set A	☐ Set A	☐ Set A
☐ Set B	☐ Set B	☐ Set B	☐ Set B	☐ Set B
☐ Neither	☐ Neither	☐ Neither	☐ Neither	☐ Neither

AR 5
Practice

Practice Exercise 5

Set A

Set B

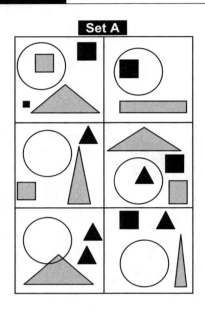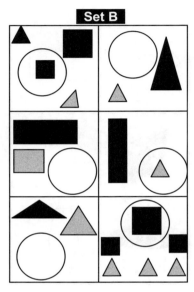

To which of the two sets above do the following shapes belong?

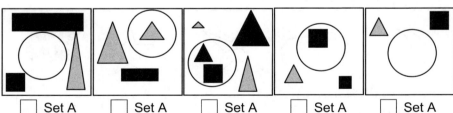

Shape 5.1	Shape 5.2	Shape 5.3	Shape 5.4	Shape 5.5
☐ Set A	☐ Set A	☐ Set A	☐ Set A	☐ Set A
☐ Set B	☐ Set B	☐ Set B	☐ Set B	☐ Set B
☐ Neither	☐ Neither	☐ Neither	☐ Neither	☐ Neither

AR 6
Practice

Practice Exercise 6

Set A

Set B

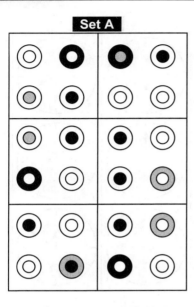
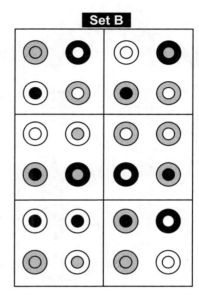

To which of the two sets above do the following shapes belong?

Shape 6.1 | **Shape 6.2** | **Shape 6.3** | **Shape 6.4** | **Shape 6.5**

☐ Set A   ☐ Set A   ☐ Set A   ☐ Set A   ☐ Set A

☐ Set B   ☐ Set B   ☐ Set B   ☐ Set B   ☐ Set B

☐ Neither   ☐ Neither   ☐ Neither   ☐ Neither   ☐ Neither

AR 7
Practice

Practice Exercise 7

Set A

Set B

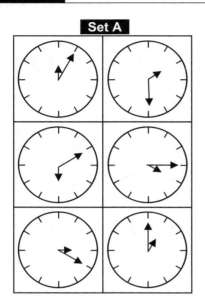
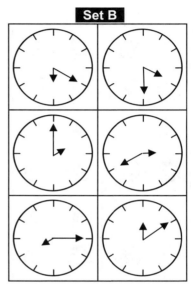

To which of the two sets above do the following shapes belong?

Shape 7.1	Shape 7.2	Shape 7.3	Shape 7.4	Shape 7.5

☐ Set A ☐ Set A ☐ Set A ☐ Set A ☐ Set A

☐ Set B ☐ Set B ☐ Set B ☐ Set B ☐ Set B

☐ Neither ☐ Neither ☐ Neither ☐ Neither ☐ Neither

| AR 8 Practice | **Practice Exercise 8** |

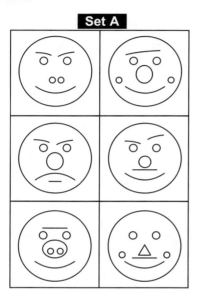 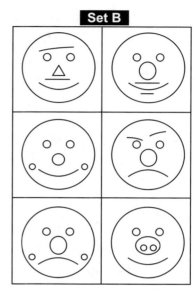

To which of the two sets above do the following shapes belong?

Shape 8.1	Shape 8.2	Shape 8.3	Shape 8.4	Shape 8.5

☐ Set A   ☐ Set A   ☐ Set A   ☐ Set A   ☐ Set A

☐ Set B   ☐ Set B   ☐ Set B   ☐ Set B   ☐ Set B

☐ Neither   ☐ Neither   ☐ Neither   ☐ Neither   ☐ Neither

AR 9
Practice

Practice Exercise 9

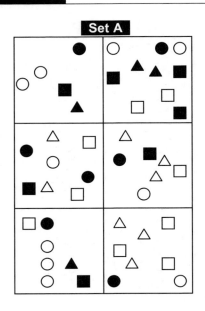

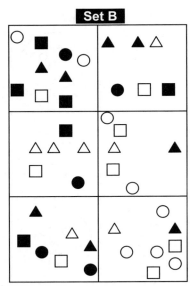

To which of the two sets above do the following shapes belong?

Shape 9.1   **Shape 9.2**   **Shape 9.3**   **Shape 9.4**   **Shape 9.5**

Set A	Set A	Set A	Set A	Set A
Set B	Set B	Set B	Set B	Set B
Neither	Neither	Neither	Neither	Neither

AR 10 Practice — Practice Exercise 10

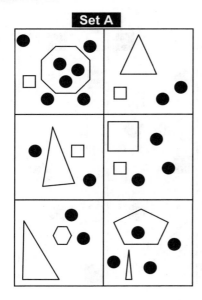

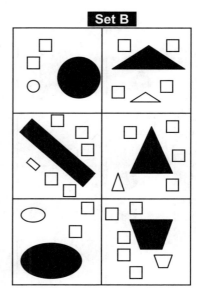

To which of the two sets above do the following shapes belong?

Shape 10.1	Shape 10.2	Shape 10.3	Shape 10.4	Shape 10.5

Set A ☐ Set A ☐ Set A ☐ Set A ☐ Set A ☐

Set B ☐ Set B ☐ Set B ☐ Set B ☐ Set B ☐

Neither ☐ Neither ☐ Neither ☐ Neither ☐ Neither ☐

AR 11
Practice

Practice Exercise 11

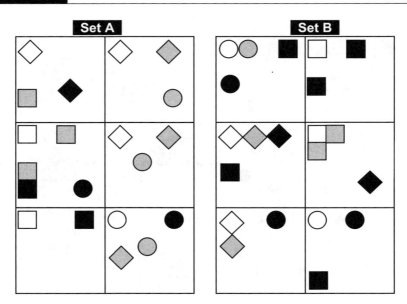

To which of the two sets above do the following shapes belong?

Shape 11.1	Shape 11.2	Shape 11.3	Shape 11.4	Shape 11.5

- [ ] Set A   [ ] Set A   [ ] Set A   [ ] Set A   [ ] Set A
- [ ] Set B   [ ] Set B   [ ] Set B   [ ] Set B   [ ] Set B
- [ ] Neither   [ ] Neither   [ ] Neither   [ ] Neither   [ ] Neither

AR 12
Practice
Practice Exercise 12

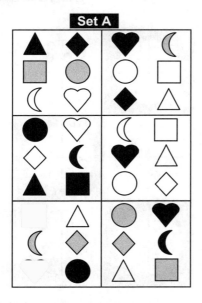 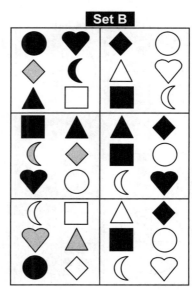

To which of the two sets above do the following shapes belong?

| Shape 12.1 | Shape 12.2 | Shape 12.3 | Shape 12.4 | Shape 12.5 |

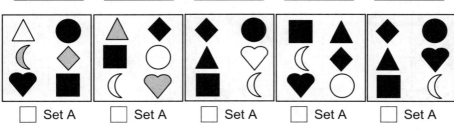

Set A	Set A	Set A	Set A	Set A
Set B	Set B	Set B	Set B	Set B
Neither	Neither	Neither	Neither	Neither

AR 13 Practice	Practice Exercise 13

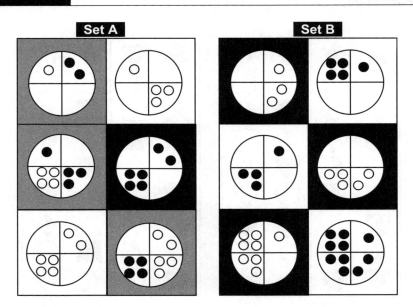

To which of the two sets above do the following shapes belong?

Shape 13.1	Shape 13.2	Shape 13.3	Shape 13.4	Shape 13.5

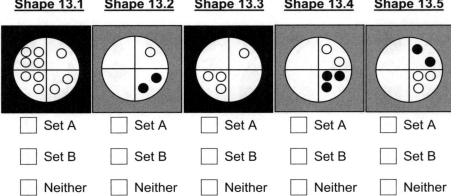

☐ Set A	☐ Set A	☐ Set A	☐ Set A	☐ Set A
☐ Set B	☐ Set B	☐ Set B	☐ Set B	☐ Set B
☐ Neither	☐ Neither	☐ Neither	☐ Neither	☐ Neither

AR 14
Practice
Practice Exercise 14

Set A   **Set B**

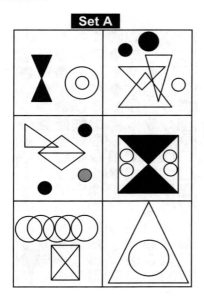
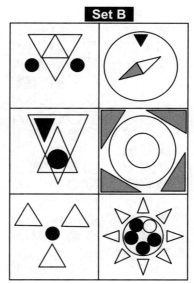

To which of the two sets above do the following shapes belong?

Shape 14.1   **Shape 14.2**   **Shape 14.3**   **Shape 14.4**   **Shape 14.5**

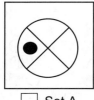

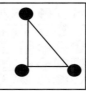

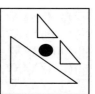

	Set A		Set A		Set A		Set A		Set A
	Set B		Set B		Set B		Set B		Set B
	Neither		Neither		Neither		Neither		Neither

AR 15
Practice

Practice Exercise 15

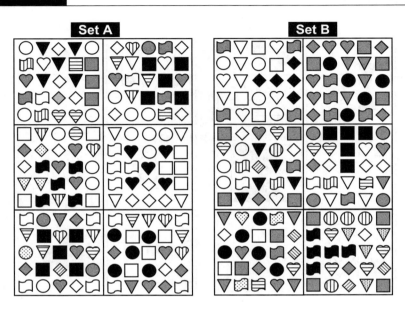

To which of the two sets above do the following shapes belong?

Shape 15.1   **Shape 15.2**   **Shape 15.3**   **Shape 15.4**   **Shape 15.5**

☐ Set A	☐ Set A	☐ Set A	☐ Set A	☐ Set A
☐ Set B	☐ Set B	☐ Set B	☐ Set B	☐ Set B
☐ Neither	☐ Neither	☐ Neither	☐ Neither	☐ Neither

AR 16 Practice	Practice Exercise 16

Set A   **Set B**

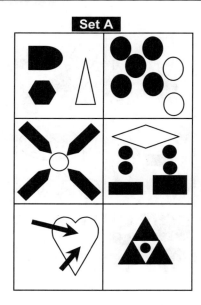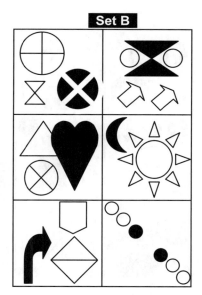

To which of the two sets above do the following shapes belong?

Shape 16.1	Shape 16.2	Shape 16.3	Shape 16.4	Shape 16.5

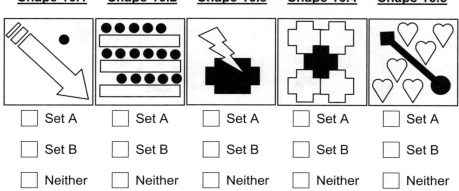

☐ Set A	☐ Set A	☐ Set A	☐ Set A	☐ Set A
☐ Set B	☐ Set B	☐ Set B	☐ Set B	☐ Set B
☐ Neither	☐ Neither	☐ Neither	☐ Neither	☐ Neither

AR 17
Practice

Practice Exercise 17

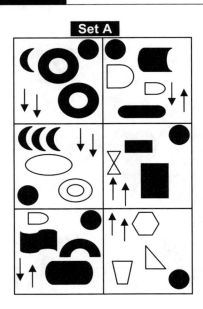

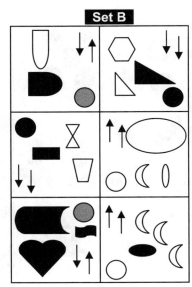

To which of the two sets above do the following shapes belong?

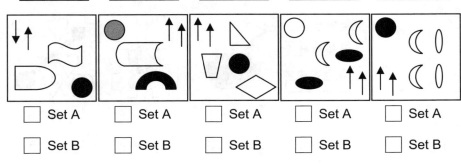

Shape 17.1

- ☐ Set A
- ☐ Set B
- ☐ Neither

Shape 17.2

- ☐ Set A
- ☐ Set B
- ☐ Neither

Shape 17.3

- ☐ Set A
- ☐ Set B
- ☐ Neither

Shape 17.4

- ☐ Set A
- ☐ Set B
- ☐ Neither

Shape 17.5

- ☐ Set A
- ☐ Set B
- ☐ Neither

AR 18 Practice — Practice Exercise 18

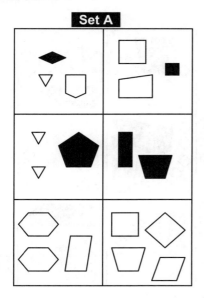

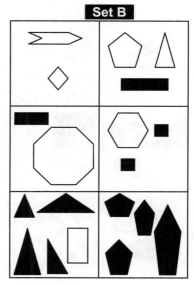

To which of the two sets above do the following shapes belong?

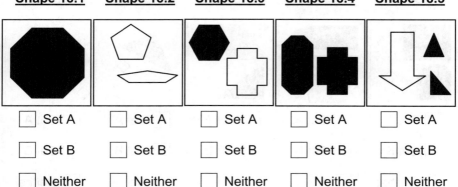

Shape 18.1	Shape 18.2	Shape 18.3	Shape 18.4	Shape 18.5
☐ Set A	☐ Set A	☐ Set A	☐ Set A	☐ Set A
☐ Set B	☐ Set B	☐ Set B	☐ Set B	☐ Set B
☐ Neither	☐ Neither	☐ Neither	☐ Neither	☐ Neither

AR 19
Practice

Practice Exercise 19

Set A

Set B

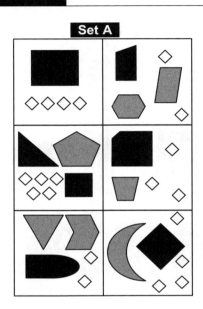
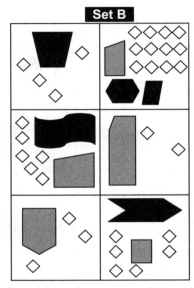

To which of the two sets above do the following shapes belong?

Shape 19.1 **Shape 19.2** **Shape 19.3** **Shape 19.4** **Shape 19.5**

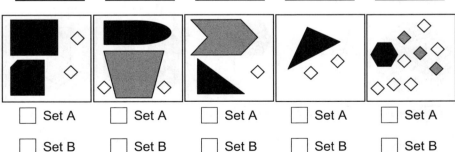

☐ Set A	☐ Set A	☐ Set A	☐ Set A	☐ Set A
☐ Set B	☐ Set B	☐ Set B	☐ Set B	☐ Set B
☐ Neither	☐ Neither	☐ Neither	☐ Neither	☐ Neither

AR 20
Practice

Practice Exercise 20

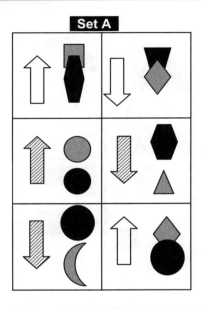

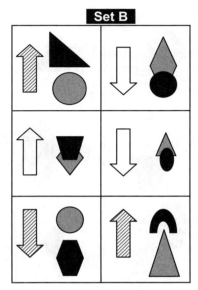

To which of the two sets above do the following shapes belong?

Shape 20.1	Shape 20.2	Shape 20.3	Shape 20.4	Shape 20.5

☐ Set A	☐ Set A	☐ Set A	☐ Set A	☐ Set A
☐ Set B	☐ Set B	☐ Set B	☐ Set B	☐ Set B
☐ Neither	☐ Neither	☐ Neither	☐ Neither	☐ Neither

AR 21
Practice

Practice Exercise 21

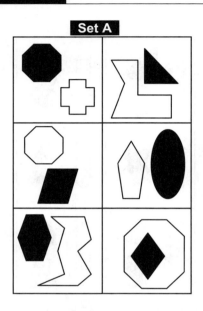

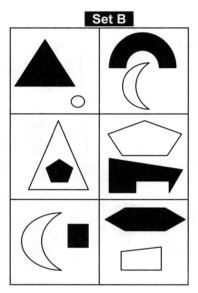

To which of the two sets above do the following shapes belong?

Shape 21.1 **Shape 21.2** **Shape 21.3** **Shape 21.4** **Shape 21.5**

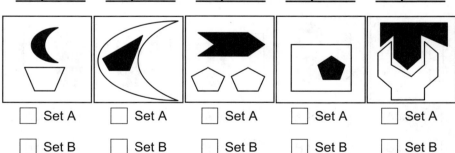

Set A	Set A	Set A	Set A	Set A
Set B	Set B	Set B	Set B	Set B
Neither	Neither	Neither	Neither	Neither

AR 22
Practice

Practice Exercise 22

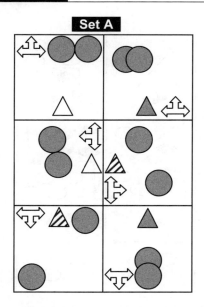

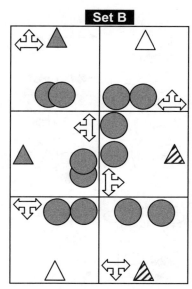

To which of the two sets above do the following shapes belong?

Shape 22.1   **Shape 22.2**   **Shape 22.3**   **Shape 22.4**   **Shape 22.5**

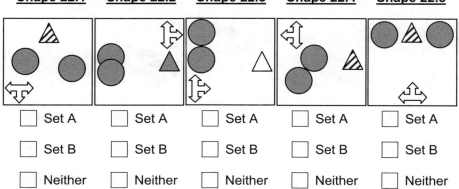

Set A	Set A	Set A	Set A	Set A
Set B	Set B	Set B	Set B	Set B
Neither	Neither	Neither	Neither	Neither

AR 23
Practice

Practice Exercise 23

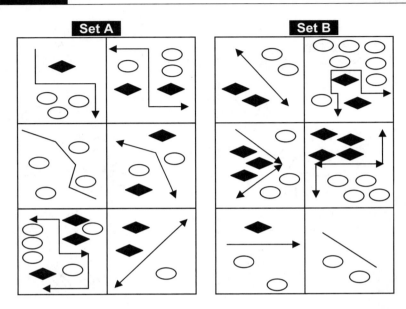

To which of the two sets above do the following shapes belong?

Shape 23.1	Shape 23.2	Shape 23.3	Shape 23.4	Shape 23.5
☐ Set A	☐ Set A	☐ Set A	☐ Set A	☐ Set A
☐ Set B	☐ Set B	☐ Set B	☐ Set B	☐ Set B
☐ Neither	☐ Neither	☐ Neither	☐ Neither	☐ Neither

AR 24
Practice

Practice Exercise 24

Set A

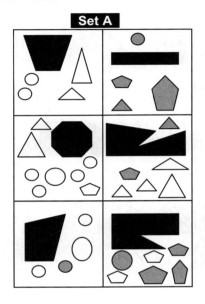

Set B

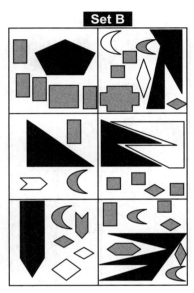

To which of the two sets above do the following shapes belong?

Shape 24.1   Shape 24.2   Shape 24.3   Shape 24.4   Shape 24.5

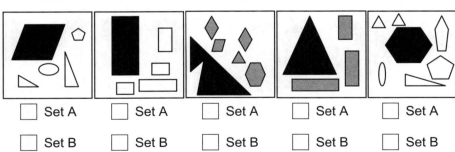

Set A	Set A	Set A	Set A	Set A
Set B	Set B	Set B	Set B	Set B
Neither	Neither	Neither	Neither	Neither

AR 25
Practice

Practice Exercise 25

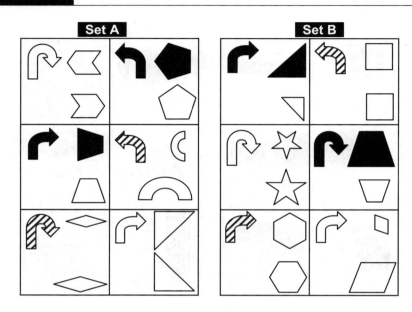

Set A

Set B

To which of the two sets above do the following shapes belong?

Shape 25.1	Shape 25.2	Shape 25.3	Shape 25.4	Shape 25.5

☐ Set A ☐ Set A ☐ Set A ☐ Set A ☐ Set A

☐ Set B ☐ Set B ☐ Set B ☐ Set B ☐ Set B

☐ Neither ☐ Neither ☐ Neither ☐ Neither ☐ Neither

AR 26 Practice

Practice Exercise 26

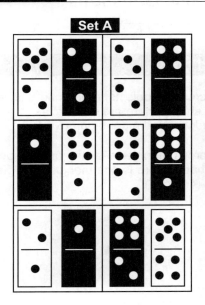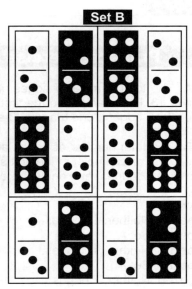

Set A   **Set B**

To which of the two sets above do the following shapes belong?

Shape 26.1   **Shape 26.2**   **Shape 26.3**   **Shape 26.4**   **Shape 26.5**

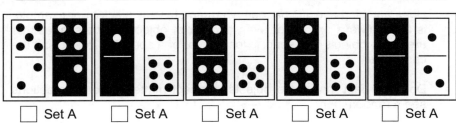

☐ Set A	☐ Set A	☐ Set A	☐ Set A	☐ Set A
☐ Set B	☐ Set B	☐ Set B	☐ Set B	☐ Set B
☐ Neither	☐ Neither	☐ Neither	☐ Neither	☐ Neither

8 Abstract Reasoning
Answers to Practice Questions

AR1 – Practice Exercise 1

Set A: The total number of edges across all objects in any one shape is equal to 13. For example, in the first shape, there are five circles (1 edge each, total 5 edges), one triangle (3 edges) and a pentagon (5 edges).

Set B: The total number of edges across all objects in any one shape is equal to 9. For example, in the first shape, there is one triangle (3 edges), two circles (2 edges) and one square (4 edges).

Answers
Shape 1.1: Neither. 10 edges.
Shape 1.2: Set A
Shape 1.3: Neither. 14 edges.
Shape 1.4: Set A
Shape 1.5: Neither. 7 edges.

Comments
Other questions that you should have asked yourself to check possible relationships (other than the basic ones) include:

- Does anything specific happen when an object is black? For example, is there always an odd or even number of objects in the shapes? Or are some objects in a specific location or of a specific size? It isn't the case here.

- Does the fact that some objects intersect matter? The intersections seem random here.

The fact that the objects in each shape are in very different combinations suggests that the relationships are not linked to the objects themselves. When you are presented with shapes which are very different, it is a good idea to check the number of sides to check a possible link. You only need to check three shapes to establish whether a pattern is present; if you find the same number then proceed to count the sides for the other shapes.

AR2 – Practice Exercise 2

Set A: There is at least one circle in each shape. All other objects have only straight edges (e.g. triangles, pentagons, squares).

Set B: There is also at least one circle in each shape, but also one object which has both straight and curved edges. There is also always one additional object with straight edges.

Answers
Shape 2.1: Neither. All curves have straight edges, but there is no circle.
Shape 2.2: Set B
Shape 2.3: Neither. No straight-edged shape and no mixed shape either.
Shape 2.4: Neither. No circle.
Shape 2.5: Neither. No circle.

Comments
The presence of a circle in each shape should be straightforward to detect at a glance. So is the presence of the mixed objects in Set B as they are in large format. This should lead you to think quickly that Set B must have at least one circle and one of the mixed objects.

At this point you must investigate whether there is a relationship with any other shapes. What we can say for Set B is that once we have excluded the circles and the big mixed object, we are left with either triangles or squares: all objects with straight edges.

You must also investigate further whether there is any relationship with the black colouring, but since Set B has two shapes which contain the same objects with a slightly different arrangement it is unlikely.

The relationship in Set A would be set to balance that in Set B in that we also have one circle at least and one object with straight edges, but no mixed object. Remember to use that "mirror" approach to derive the relationship in one set from that of the other set. It will save you a lot of time.

AR3 – Practice Exercise 3

Set A: Arrows point in all directions except towards the right.
Set B: Arrows point in all directions except towards the left.

Answers
Shape 3.1: Neither. The relationship is that there should be arrows pointing in all directions except right (Set A) or left (Set B). In 3.1, there are no downward-pointing arrows. This illustrates the need to derive the most specific relationship that you can find, i.e. in this case, not only the fact that there are no arrows pointing left or right but also the fact that there must be arrows pointing in all other directions.
Shape 3.2: Set A
Shape 3.3: Set A
Shape 3.4: Neither. Arrows pointing in all directions.
Shape 3.5: Set B

Comments
When dealing with arrows, there are a limited number of options that you can consider. Direction is the most obvious one and in this case would give you the answer. Other relationships that you would need to investigate include:

- Is the number of arrows, either in total or in a given direction, constant? For example, is there always the same number of arrows pointing upwards? In this case, the answer is no.

- Is there some relationship between two sets of arrows within a shape? For example, it could be that in one set the number of arrows pointing upwards is twice the number of arrows facing downwards (with a reverse mirror relationship for the other set). Here, the answer is no.

- Are some arrows in the same location (e.g. all arrows pointing to the left are towards the right-hand side of the shape)? This is not the case here.

AR4 – Practice Exercise 4

Set A: The rotational symmetry has an order of 2 (i.e. all objects look the same when rotated by half a turn).

Set B: The rotational symmetry has an order of 4 (i.e. all objects look the same when rotated by a quarter of a turn).

Answers

Shape 4.1: Neither. If the moon is rotated, it needs to do a full turn to look the same again.

Shape 4.2: Set A

Shape 4.3: Set A. (Note: if it did not have the line crossing in the middle, it would belong to Set B)

Shape 4.4: Neither. The rotational order is 5, i.e. it needs to rotate by a fifth of a turn to look the same.

Shape 4.5: Neither. The arrow needs to do a full turn to look the same again.

Comments

When you have single objects, the relationship is often linked to symmetry, to angles or number of sides. There are essentially two types of symmetry:

- Rotational symmetry (as above)
- Reflectional (or line) symmetry (i.e. you can fold along a line and obtain a mirror image).

All objects in Set A have two lines of reflectional symmetry according to two lines <u>except</u> the parallelogram drawn under the rectangle, which is not line-symmetrical. The only other symmetry left is therefore rotational.

In Set B, all objects have four lines of reflectional symmetry; however, this is a feature of objects that have a rotational symmetry order of 4 and therefore it amounts to the same relationship. So if this is the relationship that you have derived, then it is equally valid and will lead to the same result.

AR5 – Practice Exercise 5

Set A: All black objects can fit <u>together</u> within the white circle. This is not true of the grey objects.

Set B: All grey objects can fit <u>together</u> within the white circle. This is not true of the black objects.

Answers
Shape 5.1: Neither. The two black objects do not fit within the circle and neither does the grey object.
Shape 5.2: Set A
Shape 5.3: Set B
Shape 5.4: Neither. All black objects fit within the circle but so does the grey object.
Shape 5.5: Neither. Both the black object and the grey object fit within the circle.

Comments
This question is one which is best resolved by stepping back from the screen and looking at the two sets as a whole. Visually, you may be able to spot that the colour grey dominates Set A, and that the black colour dominates Set B.

Another clue is that the white circle appears in absolutely every single shape. Because of this it cannot be a distinguishing factor between Set A and Set B and therefore is likely to play some form of pivotal role. It may also simply be a distractor, but its omnipresence is worthy of investigation.

AR6 – Practice Exercise 6

The relationships rest on the number of white, black and grey areas, irrespective of whether they are inner circles or outer rings.

Set A: has a total number of 5 white sectors, 1 grey and 2 black.
Set B: has a total number of 3 white sectors, 3 grey and 2 black.

Answers
Shape 6.1: Set B
Shape 6.2: Set B
Shape 6.3: Neither. 4 white sectors.
Shape 6.4: Set A
Shape 6.5: Neither. 4 white sectors.

Comments
Other relationships that you would need to investigate but do not occur here include:

- Is there a specific colour or combination which appears in the same place (e.g. the top left corner outer ring is always white)?

- Do the same combinations reoccur (e.g. are black outer rings always associated with a black inner ring)?

- Do the circles follow in a certain order clockwise (e.g. is an outer-white-ring/ inner-grey-circle combination always followed by an outer-black-ring/ inner-white circle)?

- Is there a link between the numbers of each coloured circle (e.g. is the number of outer white rings always equal to or a multiple of the number of inner black rings)?

- Are the rings set out in mirror images or reverse mirror images (i.e. with grey remaining grey but black becoming white and vice versa)?

AR7 – Practice Exercise 7

The relationship in each set is linked to the result when one multiplies the number of hours shown by the hour hand by the number of minutes shown by the minute hand.

Set A: The number of hours multiplied by the number of minutes is 60 (12x5, 2x30, 6x10, 4x15, 3x20 and 1x60).

Set B: The number of hours multiplied by the number of minutes is 120 (6x20, 4x30, 2x60, 3x40, 8x15 and 12x10).

Answers
Shape 7.1: Neither. 3x5 = 15.
Shape 7.2: Neither. 9x15 = 135.
Shape 7.3: Neither. 3x30 = 90.
Shape 7.4: Set B
Shape 7:5: Neither. 9x60 = 540.

Comments
Exercises involving clocks will either be linked to the number of minutes/seconds (in which case you simply need to manipulate the numbers given to derive a relationship) or to the angles between the two hands.

AR8 – Practice Exercise 8

Each shape contains the same objects to make up two "eyes" and a mouth".

Set A: each large circle contains 7 objects.
Set B: each large circle contains 6 objects.

Answers
Shape 8.1: Set B
Shape 8.2: Set A
Shape 8.3: Set A
Shape 8.4: Set A
Shape 8.5: Set A

Comments
In this exercise, the fact that the objects within the large circle are set out to look like a face may make you lose sight of some of the more basic relationships such as the number of objects. Instead your brain will be looking naturally for a relationship based on symmetry or other factors linked to appearance, which may not be relevant. The lesson here is: do not ignore the obvious.

AR9 – Practice Exercise 9

The relationships are linked to the ability to link similar objects using a straight line without encountering another object.

Set A: The circles (regardless of their colour) are the <u>only</u> objects in each shape which can be linked by a straight line without encountering an object of a different type (e.g. triangle or square).

Set B: The triangles (regardless of their colour) are the <u>only</u> objects in each shape which can be linked by a straight line without encountering an object of a different type (e.g. circle or square).

Answers
Shape 9.1: Neither. The squares can also be linked by an uninterrupted line.
Shape 9.2: Neither. The squares can also be linked by an uninterrupted line.

Shape 9:3: Set A
Shape 9:4: Set A
Shape 9:5: Set A

Comment
The difficulty in this exercise is that there is a superposition of two concepts:

- You must be able to draw a straight line between similar objects.
- The circles or triangles must be the only objects for which this is possible.

If you identify only a partial relationship and miss out the fact that no other shapes can be linked by a straight line then you will get some of the answers wrong (though not all). Therefore, once you have found a relationship that, you feel, works, it is worth spending a few seconds extra to see whether it can be refined.

AR10 – Practice Exercise 10

Set A: The large object is white and the number of black circles is equal to the number of sides in the large object <u>minus</u> one. The remaining object is also white and can be of the same type or different type to the large object.

Set B: The large object is black, the number of white squares is equal to the number of sides <u>plus</u> one. The remaining object is white and is of the same type as the large object.

Answers
Shape 10.1: Set A
Shape 10.2: Neither. The big object is white and has 4 sides. Therefore the shape would require 3 black circles and not 5 in order to fit within Set A.
Shape 10.3: Neither. For the shape to fit within Set B, the small white circle would need to be a small parallelogram instead.
Shape 10.4: Neither. Two big objects stand out.
Shape 10.5: Set B

Comments
Too often, candidates look for relationships which are more complex than they really are. In many cases, a simple count of the number of sides is worth doing. To save time, simply count the sides in two shapes in each set to determine a possible pattern. If a pattern seems to emerge then count the rest.

AR11 – Practice Exercise 11

Both sets contain a white 'key' object in the top left corner. It is the position of the other copies of this object that are important, either horizontally, vertically or on the diagonal. The other objects are irrelevant.

Set A: Grey copies of the key object are two spaces away from the key object whilst black copies are three spaces away.

Set B: Grey copies of the key object are one space away from the key object whilst black copies are two spaces away.

Answers
Shape 11.1: Set B
Shape 11.2: Set B
Shape 11.3: Neither. The black copy is one step away. It would need to be two or three steps away to belong to any set.
Shape 11.4: Set B
Shape 11.5: Neither. The black copy is one step away, as is the grey copy. The black copy would need to be two steps away for the object to belong to Set B.

Comments
Look out for shapes with objects which are well aligned. In such cases, the relationships are often linked to their relative positions. In such cases, try to select the shapes which have some obvious features (such as the second shape of the second column in Set A, where you can clearly see that the two grey squares are two places away from the white object. This may give you an idea. In many cases, it can be difficult to determine a relationship based simply on one of the sets.

Use the fact that the relationships in both sets are of a similar nature to get ideas. For example, you may spot that in Set B the grey object is always close to the white object. Ask yourself whether there is a similar relationship in Set A. Once you have established the relationship between white and grey objects, ask yourself whether there may be a similar relationship for the black objects.

AR12 – Practice Exercise 12

Both sets have the same different shapes laid out in the same clockwise order, i.e. Triangle, Diamond, Circle, Heart, Moon and Square. The two sets differ in the relationships between the colours.

Set A:
- The Square and the Circle are always the same colour.
- The Triangle and the Heart are always of opposite colour (i.e. when one is black, the other one is white).

Set B :
- The Triangle and the Heart are always the same colour.
- The Square and the Circle are always of opposite colour (i.e. when one is black, the other one is white).

Answers
Shape 12.1: Neither. The objects are in the wrong order.
Shape 12.2: Set B
Shape 12.3: Set A
Shape 12.4: Set B
Shape 12.5: Neither. Triangle, Heart, Square and Circle are all of the same colour.

Comments
When the same objects are present in all shapes, you should watch out for the following:
- Is the object in one particular position always of the same colour or a particular type, e.g. is the top right corner shape always white or always a square? (this is not the case here)
- Is there a relationship between two objects, e.g. a black triangle always matches with a white heart? (this is the case here in Set A)
- Are the objects laid out in a certain order? (watch out in particular for clockwise orders – this is the case here)

AR13 – Practice Exercise 13

The relationships are linked to the order in which the series of dots rotates and their colours depending on the quarter in which they sit. The colour of the background is determined by the colours of the dots.

Set A:
The quarters may or may not contain dots. However, if they do, then the top left quarter only contains one, the top right quarter contains two, the bottom right quarter contains three and the bottom left quarter contains four.

All the dots within one quarter must be of the same colour, but they can have different colours between quarters. If the dots are all of the same colour then the background is of that colour. If the dots are of different colours then the background is grey.

Set B:
The number of dots also rotates clockwise, but starting from the top right quarter instead of the top left quarter. All dots must be of the same colour. The background is of the opposite colour (i.e. black if the dots are white, and white if the dots are black. Grey is not an option in Set B).

Answers
Shape 13.1: Set B
Shape 13.2: Neither. The colour pattern matches the requirement for Set A but the position of the dots does not.
Shape 13.3: Set B
Shape 13.4: Set A
Shape 13.5: Set A

Comments
In these shapes, it will get you nowhere to count the circles. The presence of several circles and the mix of colours make it difficult for the eye to pick up relationships quickly. If you are struggling to find a relationship within 30 seconds, you may want to back away from the page/screen to detach yourself from the detail. You will often find that it enables you to pick up some clues much more easily, such as – in this case – the fact that the circles are set out in a clockwise 1, 2, 3, 4 pattern, always starting from the same quadrant.

AR14 – Practice Exercise 14

The relationship is simply linked to the number of triangles versus the number of circles.

Set A: The number of triangles is equal to the number of circles.
Set B: The number of triangles is equal to the number of circles + 2.

Answers
Shape 14.1: Neither. No triangles in the shape.
Shape 14.2: Set A
Shape 14.3: Neither. Number of triangles is lower than number of circles.
Shape 14.4: Neither. Number of triangles is lower than number of circles.
Shape 14.5: Set B

Comments
Many of the shapes in this exercise are set out in a way that is designed to draw your attention towards false relationships such as a possible symmetry. In reality, the relationships are much simpler, being based on a basic count of objects. Do not let yourself be distracted by appearance unless you see a clear pattern emerging.

Also note that there are very few shapes with grey. In Set A, there is only one object which is grey. This is not enough to establish a pattern and therefore the colour of the objects has to be a distractor.

AR15 – Practice Exercise 15

In each shape, there are a total of six different types of objects. One type of object is represented 5 times (the black ones) and the other five types are represented only 4 times (appearing in various colours).

Set A: The 5 black objects are set out in an "X" pattern. The corner objects are all white (this is the only type of object which has all four white). All other objects present under different colours, with no particular pattern.

Set B: The 5 black objects form a "T" pattern (either straight or at an angle). The corner objects are the same and are all grey. This is the only type of object which has all four grey. All other objects present under different colours, with no particular pattern.

Answers

Shape 15.1: Neither. The shape does have 5 black objects in a "T" pattern as well as 4 similar grey objects in the corners, suggesting that it would belong to Set B. However, the other objects would need to be in sets of four of each of the other unused objects (i.e. hearts, diamonds, squares and flags). This particular shape only has circles and triangles.

Shape 15.2: Set B

Shape 15.3: Neither. The "X" pattern is contained within Set A, but the four corners are not all from the same white object since the top left corner is taken by one of the black objects.

Shape 15.4: Set A

Shape 15.5: Neither. The objects in the black "T" shape are not all the same.

Comments

In this exercise, there are a lot of objects to count and look at: far too many to manage in just a couple of minutes. When you have busy shapes, step away from the sets and look at them from a distance. You will spot patterns more easily. Here, like in the exam, some shapes are clearer than others e.g. those with fewer colours. Look at these first and compare them to another easier shape. Once you have an idea of a possible relationship, see if it works for the other shapes.

When there are too many objects, you may also find it easier to step back to determine a possible visual pattern (such as the X or T patterns here). If your eyes are too close to the page/screen, you run the risk of paying too much attention to some of the useless detail. In these shapes, there are a lot of distractors when, all that matters, are the corner objects and the black objects.

AR16 – Practice Exercise 16

Set A: The total number of sectors is odd. There are always more black sectors than white shapes.

Set B: The total number of sectors is even. There are always more white sectors than black sectors.

Answers

Shape 16.1: Set B

Shape 16.2: Set A
Shape 16.3: Neither. One sector of each colour so no dominance.
Shape 16.4: Neither. Odd number of sectors, with dominance of white.
Shape 16.5: Neither. Odd number of sectors, with dominance of white.

Comments

On first visual inspection, you may be able to determine quickly that Set A has a black dominance and that Set B has a white dominance. You should then count the sectors and count the sides to determine any other possible relationships. In this case you would be able to determine the odd/even relationships. Note that it is not the number of objects which counts here, but the number of sectors (so for example, the white circle with a cross within it would count as four sectors and not one object).

AR17 – Practice Exercise 17

The relationships are linked to the relative positions of the arrows and the circles, the colour of the circles in the corners and the nature of the remaining objects.

Set A: The arrows always present in pairs with one being slightly lower than the other. They are always located in one corner, with a black circle present in the diagonally opposite corner.
- If the arrows both point upwards then the remaining objects all have straight edges only.
- If the arrows both point downwards then the remaining objects all have curved edges only.
- If the arrows point in opposite directions, then the remaining objects all have a mix of curved and straight edges.

Set B: The arrows always present in pairs with one being slightly lower than the other. They are always located in one corner, with a circle present in the free corner located on the same vertical line.
- If the arrows both point upwards, then the circle is white and the remaining objects all have curved edges only.
- If the arrows both point downwards, then the circle is black and the remaining objects all have straight edges only.
- If the arrows point in different directions, then the circle is grey and the remaining objects have both straight and curved edges.

Answers

Shape 17.1: Set A
Shape 17.2: Neither. No set has the circle on the same horizontal line as the arrows.
Shape 17.3: Neither. The black circle is not in a corner.
Shape 17.4: Neither. The white circle cannot be opposite the arrows.
Shape 17.5: Neither. For Set B, the black circle requires arrows pointing downwards. In any case, even if the arrows pointed down, we would need to have all straight-edged objects in order to satisfy the relationship for Set B.

Comments

The main difficulty in this exercise is that you must exclude the circle to understand the relationships. If you exclude the circle (which is present in all the shapes) then you can see more easily that each shape has objects of different natures: straight, curved or mixed edges. The other difficulty is that, other than the colour of the circle in Set B, the colour of the other objects does not matter. This confuses things visually.

When you have objects in common between all shapes, they will either be used as a key object (i.e. they will influence other objects) or they will be used as distractors. In Set A, the black circle is a distractor, i.e. it is simply sitting there, always black and always in a corner. The arrows, however, are linked to the other objects. In Set B, the colour of the circle is linked to the directions of the arrows and therefore both are pivotal objects.

AR18 – Practice Exercise 18

Set A: The total number of edges equals 16 when counting black objects as double.
Set B: The total number of edges equals 20 when counting white objects as double.

Answers

Shape 18.1: Set A. 8 sides x 2 = 16
Shape 18.2: Set B. 2 x 5 + 2 x 5 = 20
Shape 18.3: Neither. The total number of sides is 12 + 6 = 18. Since both of the objects are of a different colour then one of the numbers will need to be doubled, which will take the number of sides way over 20.
Shape 18.4: Set B. Total number of edges = 12 + 8 = 20 in black.

Shape 18.5: Set B. 7 edges in the arrow x 2 = 14. Adding 2 x 3 sides = 6 sides for the triangles gives 20.

Comments

If counting sides does not lead you to any immediate conclusion, do not forget to allow for the colour element. In most cases (and indeed in the exam itself), the most likely relationship is that one colour will count double. If a straight count or a count based on one colour being doubled does not lead you to any conclusion then move on.

AR19 – Practice Exercise 19

Set A: All objects which have a right angle are black. Those with no right angle are grey. The number of white diamonds is equal to the number of right angles present in the coloured objects within the shape.

Set B: All objects which have a right angle are grey. Those with no right angle are black. The number of white diamonds is equal to the number of angles which are not right angles in the coloured objects within the shape.

Answers

Shape 19.1: Neither. The black objects all have right angles, which would suggest Set A. However, the number of white diamonds is equal to the number of angles which are not right angles instead of the number of right angles.

Shape 19.2: Set A

Shape 19.3: Set A

Shape 19.4: Neither. One right angle and the object is black suggests Set A. However, there are two diamonds instead of one.

Shape 19.5: Set B

AR20 – Practice Exercise 20

There is always one arrow on the left-hand side, with two other objects (one black, one grey) on its right, one being above the other.

Set A:

- If the arrow points upwards then the grey object is higher than the black object. If the arrow points downwards then the black object is higher than the grey object.

- A white arrow means that the two objects overlap, with the bottom object being above the top object.
- A shaded arrow means that the two objects do not overlap.

Set B:
- If the arrow points upwards then the black object is higher than the grey object. If the arrow points downwards then the grey object is higher than the black object.
- A white arrow means that the two objects overlap, with the black object being on top of the grey object.
- A shaded arrow means that the two objects do not overlap.

Answers
Shape 20.1: Neither. A white arrow means objects should overlap.
Shape 20.2: Set A
Shape 20.3: Neither. The black object would need to be on top of the grey object in order for the shape to belong to Set B. To belong to Set A, the black object would need to be above the grey object, with the black object being on top.
Shape 20.4: Set B
Shape 20.5: Neither. The arrow is on the right instead of the left.

Comments
Objects which feature on their own within each of the shapes are often the main drivers for the relationships within shapes. For example, in this case, the arrow is dictating through both its orientation and its colour the order and colour of the other objects.

If you identify an object which is likely to play such pivotal role, it is often best to avoid looking at all the shapes at the same time. For example, rather than looking at Set A in its entirety, start looking at the shapes which have white arrows (regardless of their orientation) and see what they have in common. Then look at the shapes which have an arrow pointing upwards (regardless of colour) and see what they have in common.

Bearing in mind that the relationships in Set A and Set B are often related, look at shapes with similar features in both sets. For example, looking at the shapes which have an upwards pointing arrow both in Set A and Set B will help you determine easily that in Set A the grey object is always above the black object whilst in Set B the reverse applies.

AR21 – Practice Exercise 21

Each shape has two objects: one black, one white.

Set A: The white object always has 4 more sides than the black object.
Set B: The black object always has 2 more sides than the white object.

Answers
Shape 21.1: Neither. The white shape has 2 more sides than the black shape.
Shape 21.2: Set B
Shape 21.3: Neither. It does have 10 white edges and 6 black edges which would suggest Set A. However, it contains 3 objects instead of the 2 contained in all shapes within Set A.
Shape 21.4: Neither. Difference between numbers of sides is only one.
Shape 21.5: Set A

Comments
The seemingly random nature of the objects (including the fact that some have angles and others don't and that some are totally separate and others within one another) suggests that the relationships is linked to the number of sides rather than any other feature.

AR22 – Practice Exercise 22

Each shape has one three-arrow object, one triangle and two circles. In all shapes:

- The set of arrows is always in a corner.
- The triangle is always in the middle alongside an edge.
- If the triangle is white then the two circles are side to side.
- If the triangle is striped then the two circles are not touching.
- If the triangle is grey then the two circles overlap.

Set A: The set of arrows points in three directions except one. The triangle is located in the middle of the edge towards which no arrow points. So, for example if the three arrows point left, down and right, then the triangle will be in the middle of the top edge of the shape. The location of the circles within the shape is random.

Set B: The triangle is located in the middle of the edge towards which the middle arrow points. So, for example if the three arrows point left, down and right, then the triangle will be in the middle of the bottom edge of the shape. The circles are always located along the edge opposite the triangle.

Answers
Shape 22.1: Set A
Shape 22.2: Set B
Shape 22.3: Set B
Shape 22.4: Neither. The triangle is striped but the circles touch.
Shape 22.5: Neither. The arrows are in the middle of the bottom side.

Comments
All objects are of a similar nature in all shapes, the only distinguishing factors being the orientation of the arrows and the location of the objects. When large arrows are present within a shape, they are often used as a pivotal object, i.e. an object that guides the others. Since arrows are primarily used for directions, it makes sense to look at the position of the other objects in relation to the directions in which the arrows are pointing.

Since all circles are grey, they are only involved either because of their location of because of their overlapping nature. By looking at the shapes which have similarly arranged circles (e.g. just touching, or overlapping) then you should be able to spot their link to the colour of the triangles.

AR23 – Practice Exercise 23

All black objects are the same and all white objects are the same.

Set A:
- The number of black objects equals the number of arrowheads.
- The number of white objects equals the number of straight lines.
- The objects are spread randomly within the shape.

Set B:
- The number of black objects equals the number of arrowheads.
- The number of white objects equals the number of straight lines + 1.
- The white and black objects are separated by the straight lines forming a boundary.

Answers

Shape 23.1: Set A

Shape 23.2: Neither. The number of black objects is greater than number of arrowheads.

Shape 23.3: Neither. The numbers of white and black objects satisfy the relationship for Set B. However, the objects are randomly set out instead of being separated on each side of the boundary.

Shape 23.4: Set B

Shape 23.5: Neither. The shape would meet the criteria for Set B if the two white objects were on the same side of the line.

Comments

When a shape contains many arrows, the relationships are either linked to the directions of the arrows (e.g. they are all pointing in the same direction) or they are used as a pivotal shape with the other objects in the shape being linked, as is the case here, to the number arrows or arrow heads.

Look out for shapes that have similar features as they provide valuable clues. For example, two shapes in Set A have 3 white ovals but have 1 and 2 black diamonds respectively. The only difference between the two is the number of arrow heads. Similarly in Set B, the top two shapes both have 2 black diamonds but the second shape has many more white ovals (which can be linked to the more complex set of straight lines).

AR24 – Practice Exercise 24

In both sets there is only one black object and the number of other objects is equal to the number of sides (and therefore angles) in the black object.

Set A: The black object has an even number of sides. All other objects (white or grey) have an odd number of sides. The number of grey objects equals the number of right angles in the black object. All other objects are white (and therefore their number equals the number of angles in the black object which are not right angles).

Set B: The black object has an odd number of sides. All other objects (white or grey) have an even number of sides. The number of white objects equals the number of right angles in the black object. All other objects are grey (and therefore their number equals the number of angles on the black object which are not right angles).

Answers
Shape 24.1: Set A
Shape 24.2: Neither. The colour pattern suits Set B. However, the white objects have an even number of sides, whilst they should have an odd number of sides (i.e. be triangles, pentagons, etc.).
Shape 24.3: Neither. The grey shapes have a mix of even and odd number of sides (e.g. triangle and diamond).
Shape 24.4: Set B
Shape 24:5: Set A

Comments
The presence of a large black object should alert you to the fact that it plays a pivotal role (the exercise would be too easy if there simply had to be a large black object!). Number of sides and angles usually play a sizeable role in the relationships within each set.

AR25 – Practice Exercise 25

Each set consists of three objects: one arrow and two other objects of a similar nature, though not always of the same colour or size. The size and colour of the objects is dictated by the colour of the arrow.

In all cases, the three objects are located in all but the bottom left corner and the object in the bottom right corner is always white. The shape of the object in the top right corner is taken as the shape of the object below it, rotated according to the direction of the arrow. So an arrow pointing to the right means that the object in the top right corner is equal to the object in the bottom right corner rotated 90 degrees clockwise, whilst a left-pointing arrow indicates a rotation of 90 degrees anti-clockwise. A "U-turn" arrow means that the object is rotated 180 degrees.

Set A:
▪ A white arrow means that the two other objects have the same colour and same size.
▪ A black arrow means that the two objects have the same size but the top object is black.

- A striped arrow means that the top object is white but of smaller size than the bottom object.

Set B:
- A white arrow means that both objects are white but the top object is of a smaller size.
- A black arrow means that the top object is black and is of greater size than the bottom object.
- A striped arrow means that both objects are white and of the same size.

Answers
Shape 25.1: Set A
Shape 25.2: Neither. The star is not rotated.
Shape 25.3: Set A
Shape 25.4: Set B
Shape 25.5: Neither. The black object is smaller than the white object, which fits the profile of neither set in the presence of a black arrow.

Comments
The presence of an arrow in each shape (with different orientations and colours) indicates that it is likely to play a central role in defining the other shapes. You can see clearly that the other two objects are of the same type but in different positions and colours.

To facilitate your task of identifying the relationship within each shape, avoid looking at all the shapes at the same time. Take all the shapes which have an arrow pointing towards the right and see whether you can identify a trend. Similarly look at all the shapes which have a white/striped arrow and see if you can spot similarities.

When several parameters come into play (e.g. colour and orientation), fix one of these parameters by selecting all the shapes that satisfy it (e.g. by selecting all white arrows) and see how the other parameter influences the shapes.

AR26 – Practice Exercise 26

Each shape contains two dominoes, one of which is black and the other one white. The relationships are linked to the orientation of the dominoes and the total number of dots on each domino.

Set A:
In each domino, the higher number of dots is at the top and the lower number of dots is at the bottom. The domino with the lower total number of dots is black.

Set B:
In each domino, the higher number of dots is at the bottom and the lower number of dots is at the top. The domino with the higher total number of dots is black.

Answer
Shape 26.1: Set A
Shape 26.2: Neither. Higher number of dots is not always at the top or the bottom.
Shape 26.3: Set B
Shape 26.4: The higher number of dots is at the bottom, suggestive of Set B. However, the domino with the lower total number of dots is black.
Shape 26.5: Neither. The higher number of dots is at the top and at the bottom respectively.

Comments
In the same way that, when you have clocks, the answer usually has to do either with the angle between the two hands or with the result of adding up or multiplying the numbers pointed to by the two hands, when you have dominoes the relationships are fairly limited. You would need to look at the following:

- where the larger or smaller number of dots are positioned.
- the total number of dots of each domino, across the top or the bottom and on the diagonals.
- the relationship between two sets of dots (e.g. is the top number of dots always one more than the bottom number of dots?).

VERBAL REASONING

TIPS & TECHNIQUES

+

96
PRACTICE QUESTIONS & ANSWERS

9 Verbal Reasoning
Format, Purpose & Key Techniques

FORMAT

The verbal reasoning test consists of 11 text passages which deal with a wide range of topics. Those topics are generic and do not necessarily relate to medicine. The text passages usually contain 200 to 350 words and may take different forms including newspaper articles, instruction manuals or even complaint letters. For each of the 11 text passages, you are given 4 statements. For each statement, you will be asked to determine whether that statement is "True", "False", or "Can't tell" based on the information provided in the text.

EXAMPLE

Text
Some common foods can interfere with medications. Grapefruit juice is specifically in the line of fire. Drinking it could indeed dangerously worsen the side effects of some drugs because it facilitates their absorption into the system. In particular, the interaction of grapefruit juice with simvastatin and, to a lesser extent, with atorvastatin (two anti-cholesterol drugs) can lead to severe muscular problems. With transplant anti-rejection drugs, such as tacrolimus and cyclosporin, the kidneys are endangered. Finally, with cisapride, prescribed for severe gastric reflux, there are risks of severe cardiac arrhythmia.

Question
Patients taking simvastatin are likely to experience more severe side effects than patients taking atorvastatin.

Answer: CAN'T TELL
The text states that grapefruit juice interacts with atorvastatin to a lesser extent than with simvastatin. This does not mean that simvastatin gives more severe side effects than atorvastatin. The text does not deal with the side effects of the two drugs in normal circumstances and therefore we cannot conclude based on what is contained in the text.

The time given at the exam to answer all 44 questions is 22 minutes (1 minute to read the instructions and 21 minutes to answer). On average, you therefore have just under 2 minutes per text or 30 seconds per question.

PURPOSE

The purpose of the verbal reasoning test is to determine whether you are able to comprehend information and interpret it in a meaningful way. In Medicine, this is an important skill that you will need to use in many contexts. For example:

- Throughout your medical career, you will be required to read journals and interpret the findings presented in research papers. In some cases, you will need to draw the lessons from such papers so that you can apply them to your own clinical practice. It is therefore crucial that you draw the right conclusions.

- The study of Medicine and putting it into effective practice involves the learning and understanding of what factors cause or affect a disease, for which you will need to ensure that you are able to draw the correct conclusions from the information at your disposal. For example, a study may uncover the fact that most patients with lung cancer are also regular drinkers; however, this does not necessarily mean that alcohol causes lung cancer. Indeed, it could be that most people who smoke also happen to drink.

- As a doctor, you will gain much information from talking to your patients. It is particularly important that you make decisions based on the information available to you rather than by jumping to the wrong conclusions either because you have misunderstood what you were being told or because you made assumptions.

The verbal reasoning test is therefore primarily a logic test as well as a test of your ability to interpret information based on known facts.

KEY TECHNIQUES

In the verbal reasoning test, there are a number of difficulties that you must be aware of and that you must practise to overcome:

Practise reading the text quickly and efficiently
Since you have under 2 minutes to read the text and answer all four questions, you will not have enough time to read any 300-word text in detail. You should therefore practise to gather all important information quickly.

Very often, a question will refer to information contained in a specific paragraph or sentence of the text only and not the whole text. In the example discussed on the previous page, the question could be answered simply by looking at the sentence *"In particular, the interaction of grapefruit juice with simvastatin and, to a lesser extent, with atorvastatin (two anti-cholesterol drugs) can lead to severe muscular problems"*. Therefore, when you read the text for the first time, you may want to simply scan through it to identify the different topics that it addresses. For example, the text on the previous page may be categorised as follows:

- Generalities on grapefruit juice
- Cholesterol drugs
- Transplant drugs
- Gastric drugs.

When you read the question, you can then refer to the relevant portion of text in more detail. This way, you only read in detail what you really need to read, which can save you a lot of time considering that many of the texts contain information that is never used in the questions.

You may still encounter questions which require information to be gathered from different paragraphs and may therefore take up a lot of time to answer; but the time you will have saved on the more straightforward questions should enable you to spend a bit more time on these.

Focus on the text and ignore what you know through other means
Some texts may deal with issues with which you are familiar or may be based on facts or assumptions that contradict information that you know through other sources. In some cases, the text might give information that you know to be inaccurate. Whatever your prior knowledge, the text is the only source of information that you should consider.

Learn to interpret keywords that are likely to influence the answers
Both the text and the questions may contain phrases which could be easily overlooked when read quickly (such as "may", "might", "would", "could",

"can", "only", "the most", "the least", "commonly") and could switch the answer from "True" or "False" to "Can't tell". In particular:

► "Can" means that it is possible for an event to take place, even if it is not frequently. For example, sharks can eat human beings. It does not mean that they do it often; it does not mean that all sharks do it; and it does not mean either that it has ever happened. "May", "Might" and "Could" also mean that an event is possible without any reference to frequency or probability. For example, prolonged exposure to sun rays may lead to skin cancer. It is simply possible (i.e. it has probably happened to some people but that is as far as you can conclude).

► "Commonly" and "Frequently" suggest that an event is not an unusual occurrence. It does not mean that it happens all the time or to everyone, though it implies that it would happen in a majority of cases (i.e. over 50%). It is simply something that one should be expecting to happen in many instances under common conditions. For example, high cholesterol is commonly associated with either poor diet or family history, i.e. these would be considered two important factors that would affect most people.

► "Many" suggests a large number but not necessarily a majority. For example, many of newborn babies are male. It does not mean that the majority of newborn babies are male. "Many" therefore relates to a number rather than a proportion. "Most" or "The majority", however, refer to a proportion. Depending on the context, 'most' may mean either that it applies to over 50% of the population or sometimes an overwhelming majority, i.e. "most people who replied to the survey were from London" suggests a large percentage, though one cannot really say for sure. The use of "most" also suggests that some people do not fall into that category.

► "Unlikely" refers to something that has a probability which is too low to be considered seriously. For example, you are unlikely to be eaten by a shark in the Mediterranean if none of the sharks in that sea have ever bitten anyone or if these sharks are vegetarian, but it is not completely impossible. It is just highly improbable.

▶ "Cannot" and "Impossible" refer to events that can never happen, i.e. it is simply not possible. For example, men cannot fly without the help of technology. In practice, there are very few things that are truly impossible; so if a question is asking you to comment on the fact that a particular event cannot take place, double-check that the answer should not be "can't tell" instead. In particular, the fact that something has never happened before or has an extremely low chance of occurring does not mean that it is impossible. You see that a lot in court cases; for example, the probability that three babies by the same mother die of cot death has an extremely low probability but one can't tell for sure that it cannot happen.

▶ "Average" is a word that occurs often in the texts used in the exam. Usually the text will give an average and the statement in the question will ask you whether the average figure can be applied to any particular individual. For example, the text could say: "The average unemployment rate across all UK counties was 3% in 2007." The question would then state "Unemployment in Surrey was 3% in 2007", which we cannot confirm either way since the only figure we are given is an average across the country.

Questions containing average can cause a particular problem. For example, in the example above, consider the question "Some counties had an unemployment rate under 3% in 2007." One could reasonably state that, since the figure of 3% is an average, some counties would have a rate below 3% and others a rate above 3%, and that therefore the statement is true. However, there is also a (very remote) possibility that all counties have an unemployment rate of exactly 3%, in which case the average would still be 3% but the statement would be false. It is of course highly improbable but still possible. In the absence of conclusive information, I would suggest that you opt for "can't tell" as this would be the absolutely correct answer.

Practise the key logic rules

The verbal reasoning test is a test of comprehension and logic, i.e. can you deduce the right information from what you are given. There are two logic rules which are often used in the exam to create questions:

> ► Rule 1: If A → B, then you always have (non-B) →(non-A).
> ► Rule 2: If A → B, then (non-A) does not always imply (non-B).

Consider the following statement: "All shoes made by the ABC Company are made of real leather." We can conclude from this statement that shoes which are not made of real leather cannot come from the ABC Company (Rule 1). However, we cannot conclude from the statement that all shoes which are not made by the ABC Company are not made of real leather (Rule 2). Indeed the statement does not exclude the fact that other companies may also make shoes with real leather.

Differentiate link and causation

The text may present facts which seem related, may be linked but do not necessarily have a direct cause and effect relationship. For example, consider this text: "Scientists have found that the vast majority patients of patients who contracted a liver disease had also been heavy smokers throughout their life." This indicates that there is a relationship between smoking and liver disease but you should be careful not to over-extrapolate. Consider the following statements:

Q: Smoking causes liver disease.
A: Can't tell. Based on the text, this is a possibility, but it is also possible that smoking is associated with other behaviours which lead to liver disease. For example, it may be that all heavy drinkers also happen to be heavy smokers.

Q: Smokers are more likely to develop liver disease than non-smokers.
A: Can't tell. It depends on the ratio of smokers and non-smokers in the general population. So, for example, let's say that 90% of those with liver disease were found to be heavy smokers, but that, in the general population, 90% were heavy smokers anyway; then the statistics would not be that meaningful. However, if only 20% of people in the overall population smoked, this would indicate that smokers are more likely to develop liver disease (although, as we have seen above, this may not necessarily be caused by the smoking itself, but other associated factors).

Such reasoning forms the basis of numerous questions in the test and provides an opportunity for the examiners to confuse you with statements which appear true but are in fact ambiguous. With a little bit of practice you will acquire the necessary mental agility to be able to manipulate these concepts confidently and quickly in the exam.

Answer all questions and don't be afraid of the "can't tell" option

The UKCAT is not negatively marked, i.e. you are not penalised for a wrong answer, so it is important that you tick an option, even if you are unsure. By ticking any box, you have one chance out of three to get it right. By ticking none, you are guaranteed to score nil on that question.

If you struggle with one question, it may be worth leaving it and coming back to it later on. You may get a bright idea in the meantime and, by taking a step back, you may read the text in a different light next time round.

Candidates usually find it difficult to tick the "can't tell" answer. Psychologically they may feel uncomfortable at not being able to settle on a definite answer and may be constantly worried about missing something obvious. Overall, it is easier for an examiner to write questions which have an ambiguous answer than to write questions which have a definite answer and do not appear too obvious. On balance, therefore, there ought to be more questions to which the answer is "can't tell" than the other two options. If you are really stuck on an answer, I would therefore suggest that you tick the "can't tell" box as it may have a higher probability of being the right answer (in fact, the fact that you are struggling with it in the first place may be an indication that the answer cannot actually be concluded from the text).

10 Verbal Reasoning Practice Questions

This section contains 12 texts, for which there are 8 different questions, hence a total of 96 practice questions. This is equivalent to over two full exams. These questions are designed to help you develop an awareness of the different techniques and tips mentioned in the previous section and, as such, we have therefore included more questions per text than you would anticipate being asked to answer in the exam.

If you have already practised for verbal reasoning exercises through other means, you may wish to practise these questions in real time, in which case you should aim to complete each set of 8 questions in less than 4 minutes (ideally under 3.5 minutes).

If, however, you prefer to use these 96 practice questions to develop your awareness of the various difficulties that you may encounter throughout the verbal reasoning test and to build up your skills and confidence, I would suggest that you take your time to do the first three or four exercises, checking the answers as you go along. As you progress towards the latter exercises, you should try to answer questions more quickly: the aim being to be able to answer each set of 8 questions in less than 4 minutes by the time you get to Practice Exercises 9 and 10.

The answers to all questions, together with explanations, can be found from page 176 onwards.

Once you have practised answering all 96 questions, you should be ready to confront the mock exam which features at the back of this book and replicates the actual exam's format (i.e. 11 texts, 4 questions each). You may want to wait until you have practised all sections in this book before going ahead with the mock exam.

VR 1 Practice	Financial Crisis

TEXT

The 2008 financial crisis was caused by a number of factors which can be difficult for a lay member of the public to understand. At the source of the crisis is the fact that a number of US banks had offered mortgages to so-called "sub-prime" customers (i.e. usually less well-off individuals with a high credit risk) without checking that the customers could actually afford to repay the loans. The bank had then sold the debt to other banks around the world, meaning that almost every bank in the world owned a share of these mortgages, with some owning a bigger share than others. When a large proportion of these "sub-prime" customers failed to repay some of their loans, all exposed banks started experiencing difficulties, having lent money that could not be repaid. This caused a domino effect and a major financial crisis, which included the nationalisation of Northern Rock, the collapse of American investment institutions such as Lehman Brothers, followed by the merger of Merrill Lynch with Bank of America and then the merger of HBOS with Lloyds TSB in the UK. Some commentators have said that bankers' greed was a contributor to the problem.

As if a global crisis wasn't enough, public confidence was also under-mined by an alleged pyramid scheme fraud by a prominent American fin-ancier. This $50bn alleged fraud consisted of taking money from unsus-pecting rich individuals, promising high returns. As new investors paid money into the scheme, the older investors were being paid interest or dividends using the new money, and so on. As it became increasingly dif-ficult to find new money from new investors to pay existing investors and as the old investors started to want their initial investment back, the scheme came apart and the financier had no option but to admit that there was a problem and was arrested. The alleged scam worked on an exclu-sive basis, i.e. only those who were invited could invest. This created a false sense of security which encouraged very prominent individuals, in-cluding bankers, to become victims. Pyramid schemes are non-sustainable models which involve enrolling new members and rewarding the members with money being paid by new members. They clearly ex-ploit the greed and gullibility of those who are easily attracted by high re-turns. Such schemes are illegal in many countries, including the US and the UK.

PRACTICE QUESTIONS

5/8   62.5%

Q1.1   The HBOS-Lloyds TSB merger could have been avoided if Lehman Brothers had not collapsed.

☐ True   ☐ False   ☑ Can't tell   ✓

Q1.2   The fact that international banks were linked to the American market by owning a share of the sub-prime debt played a key role in the 2008 financial crisis.

☑ True   ☐ False   ☐ Can't tell   ✓

Q1.3   If bankers had not been so greedy, there would have been no financial crisis.

☐ True   ☑ False   ☐ Can't tell   ✗

Q1.4   The 2008 financial crisis has its origin in the US.

☑ True   ☐ False   ☐ Can't tell   ✓

Q1.5   Pyramid schemes do not exist in the UK.

☐ True   ☐ False   ☑ Can't tell   ✓

Q1.6   The alleged fraud was one of the key triggers of the financial crisis.

☐ True   ☐ False   ☑ Can't tell   ✗

Q1.7   The American financier involved in the alleged fraud made a personal gain of $50bn.

☐ True   ☐ False   ☑ Can't tell   ✓

Q1.8   All pyramid schemes will fail eventually.

☐ True   ☐ False   ☑ Can't tell   ✗

VR 2 Practice	Global Warming

TEXT

There is considerable debate about the nature and causes of global warming. A large proportion of politicians believe that global warming is primarily a man-made problem and that each country should make every effort possible to reduce its carbon emissions. As a result, a range of carbon emission reduction measures are being introduced including: encouraging people to use less energy by switching to low-energy light bulbs and switching off unnecessary appliances; and reducing the number of unnecessary car journeys to the bare minimum and encouraging people to switch to public transport. Others believe that the UK is unlikely to make much of a difference since the biggest contributors to carbon emissions are countries such as China, who are refusing to take any remedial action. Others, still, believe that global warming is part of the Earth's natural cycle and that any action taken is bound to have little effect on the planet.

So, what level of global warming is anticipated for the forthcoming years? Scientists have studied several scenarios which were integrated within climate forecasting models. Assuming that no substantial change takes place, the forecast for the next century includes a rise in the average world temperature of between 1.4 and 5.8 °C and a reduction of the ice cap in the northern hemisphere, whereas in Antarctica (i.e. in the southern hemisphere) the melting of the ice cap would be more than offset by heavier snow falls, with the snow then freezing over the existing layer of ice. Sea levels are expected to increase by between 9cm and 88cm. By the end of the 21st century, the average sea level should have risen by between 18cm and 59cm. Some scientists predict that the planet's temperature rise caused by humans should continue after the year 2100. The rise in sea level should also continue for millennia after stabilisation of the climate.

Africa is especially vulnerable because of existing pressures on its ecosystems and its low capacity to adapt to change. On all continents, water supply and the threat of flooding in coastal areas will cause problems. On the other hand, areas of the world which are further away from the equator may see an increase in agricultural productivity and colder regions will see their heating needs reduced.

PRACTICE QUESTIONS

4/c = 50%

Q2.1   Switching to low-energy bulbs and encouraging people to use public transport will reduce global warming.

☐ True   ☐ False   ☑ Can't tell   ✗

Q2.2   Those who believe that global warming is a natural phenomenon also believe that there is no need to take any action.

☐ True   ☐ False   ☑ Can't tell   ✗

Q2.3   China produces the majority of carbon emissions on Earth.

☐ True   ☐ False   ☑ Can't tell   ✓

Q2.4   Global warming is used as an excuse by politicians to reduce the number of cars on the roads.

☐ True   ☑ False   ☐ Can't tell   ✗

Q2.5   In the 21st century, the sea level in Britain is projected to rise by no more than 59cm.

☐ True   ☐ False   ☑ Can't tell   ✓

Q2.6   The Antarctica ice cap is expected to grow over the 21st century.

☑ True   ☐ False   ☐ Can't tell   ✓

Q2.7   Some countries will experience no negative impact from global warming.

☑ True   ☐ False   ☐ Can't tell   ✗

Q2.8   Over the 21st century, some countries may experience a rise in temperature of over 5.8°C.

☐ True   ☐ False   ☑ Can't tell   ✓

155

VR 3 Practice	Free Museum Entry

TEXT

In 2001, the government reintroduced free entry into museums in England, Scotland and Wales, preferring instead to fund museums through governmental subsidies and Heritage Lottery Fund grants. The following year, the number of visitors increased by an average of 70%, with museums such as the V&A registering an increase of 111%.

In addition, a piece of research undertaken by Sara Selwood at City University showed that the museums which saw the biggest increase in visitor figures were also those which had opened new facilities or which had refurbished their facilities in addition to introducing free admission. Some of the increase is due to the same people who previously paid now visiting museums more often and efforts are therefore being made to broaden the appeal of museums to a wider population. As a result of this free entry policy, some independent museums, who continued charging, have seen a decline in numbers of visitors. The policy is seen as unfair competition. There is also a perception that the subsidies are mostly directed at the already wealthy London museums, and do little to encourage museums in the regions.

In 2007, the Department for Culture, Media and Sport (DCMS) announced that the free museum entry policy would be continued at least for another 3 years. Originally, the DCMS had been asked to prepare for a 5% cut in its budget, though the Chancellor, Alistair Darling, later promised that he would increase the department's funding from £1.68 billion in the 2007-2008 financial year to £2.21 billion in 2010-11. Many fear though that, in view of the current financial crisis and of the impending Olympic Games, the Arts will be placed on the backburner whilst the government addresses more pressing priorities.

The Conservative Party has developed plans to scrap free entry to museums if it came to power, arguing that allowing museums to set their own entry fees would lead to an improvement in the service they offer. This point of view is likely to anger many members of the public, although perhaps not the 40% of UK residents who, according to a recent poll, seem to be unaware of the existence of the free-entry policy.

PRACTICE QUESTIONS

-/8   25 %

Q3.1 The only impact of the "free-entry" policy has been to encourage people who already went to museums to go more often.

☑ True   ☐ False   ☐ Can't tell ✗

Q3.2 Some museums have seen an increase in visitor numbers of less than 70%.

☐ True   ☐ False   ☑ Can't tell ✗

Q3.3 Only the big London museums seem to have benefited from the free-entry policy.

☑ True   ☐ False   ☐ Can't tell ✗

Q3.4 The increase in visitor numbers is solely due to the free-entry policy.

☐ True   ☐ False   ☑ Can't tell ✓

Q3.5 Granting free museum entry to the public had never been attempted before.

☐ True   ☑ False   ☐ Can't tell ✓

Q3.6 The DCMS's budget will increase by £530 million over 3 years.

☑ True   ☐ False   ☐ Can't tell ✗

Q3.7 The 2012 Olympics will put an end to the free-entry policy.

☐ True   ☑ False   ☐ Can't tell ✗

Q3.8 A fee-paying entry policy is fairer to small museums.

☑ True   ☐ False   ☐ Can't tell ✗

VR 4 Practice	EEC, EU, EURO

TEXT

The European Economic Community (EEC) was set up in 1957 by the following countries: Belgium, France, Germany, Italy, Luxembourg and the Netherlands. The UK joined the EEC in 1973. The Maastricht Treaty of 1993 abolished the EEC and replaced it with the European Union (EU). At the time, the EU comprised the same countries as the EEC, but now includes 27 independent sovereign countries (also known as member states). The main EU institutions are the European Commission, which resides in Brussels (Belgium), and the European Parliament, which sits in Strasbourg (France). The Euro was adopted as the EU's official currency in 1999, though coins and bank notes were not produced until 2002. Fifteen EU countries, collectively known as the Eurozone, have adopted it. In addition, 11 non-EU countries have also adopted the Euro as official currency, including Monaco, the Vatican and Andorra. Sweden and the UK have both declined to join the Euro for the time being.

The UK has adopted a "wait-and-see policy". Arguments in favour of joining the Euro are numerous. By reducing exchange rate uncertainty for UK businesses and tourists, everyone would benefit from lower transaction costs. Adopting the Euro would also encourage greater competition across borders, enabling UK customers to compare prices directly with their neighbours and purchase goods accordingly. On the other hand, adopting the Euro would bring its fair share of problems. For a start, UK interest rates would be set by the European Central Bank in Frankfurt (Germany), which sets interest rates for the whole Eurozone. It has long been argued that the UK economy is more in line with US economy than with European economy and that therefore it needs to keep closer links with US interest rates than European interest rates. In December 2008, the Bank of England was able to reduce UK interest rates drastically in an attempt to boost the UK economy; this would not have been possible had the UK adopted the Euro.

With all this in mind, the most powerful argument against the Euro in the UK is the fact that UK citizens are reluctant to relinquish yet more power to Brussels and to lose their identity in an ever-expanding Europe.

PRACTICE QUESTIONS

$s/s = 62.5\%$

Q4.1 Monaco is part of the Eurozone.

☐ True   ☑ False   ☐ Can't tell ✓

Q4.2 All original EEC countries are currently in the EU.

☐ True   ☑ False   ☐ Can't tell ✗

Q4.3 All EU institutions are located either in France or in Belgium.

☐ True   ☐ False   ☑ Can't tell ✗

Q4.4 Neither Sweden nor the UK intend to adopt the Euro.

☑ True   ☐ False   ☐ Can't tell ✗

Q4.5 If the UK entered the Eurozone, the Bank of England would lose the power to set interest rates.

☑ True   ☐ False   ☐ Can't tell ✓

Q4.6 The UK would benefit more from adopting the US Dollar as its currency than from adopting the Euro.

☐ True   ☐ False   ☑ Can't tell ✓

Q4.7 Andorra is not an independent sovereign country.

☐ True   ☐ False   ☑ Can't tell ✓

Q4.8 If the UK adopted the Euro as official currency then the Bank of England would cease to exist.

☐ True   ☐ False   ☑ Can't tell ✓

| VR 5 Practice | Coq au Vin & Quiche Lorraine |

TEXT

"Coq au Vin" is a traditional French dish whose main ingredients are red wine, lardons, onion and occasionally garlic. The word "coq" means "rooster". Traditional recipes use older roosters to produce a richer broth; however, roosters are not easily found and can be tough to eat. Consequently most home cooks use chicken as a substitute. Lardons are frequently used in French cooking and consist of thick slices of pork belly cut in cubes or thick strips. They are often smoked and are a main ingredient for a wide range of dishes including Quiche Lorraine. Although they can be found in some UK supermarkets, lardons are in sparse supply and thick bacon can be used as a substitute. However, bacon is not as fatty as lardons and therefore may taste drier. The original recipe uses the bird's blood, which is added at the end to produce a thick black colour. The faint-hearted leave the blood out, though it produces a less rich sauce.

Quiche Lorraine is a dish that dates back to the 16th century, and consisted of an egg, cream and lardon mix on a crust of bread dough. Because of its primarily vegetarian ingredients, it was historically considered a somehow unmanly dish, hence the expression "real men don't eat quiche". There is controversy as to whether cheese formed part of the original dish (although the locals believe it didn't, some food historians do). Today, the Quiche Lorraine is not always served with cheese.

Its name comes from the German "Kuchen", meaning "cake", with "Lorraine" signifying that it comes from the Lorraine region in Eastern France. Lorraine, a region bordering Belgium, Germany and Luxembourg, was first taken by France in 1648, together with the Alsace region was annexed by the Germans in 1871, and handed back to the French in 1918 following WWI. Its symbol is the Mirabelle plum (a yellow cousin of the greengage), which is often used to make pastries and to make a very refined liqueur.

PRACTICE QUESTIONS $5/8 = 62.5\%$

Q5.1   Bacon is an essential ingredient of Coq au Vin.

☐ True   ☑ False   ☐ Can't tell ✓

Q5.2   Bacon can be used as a substitute for lardons in Quiche Lorraine.

☐ True   ☐ False   ☑ Can't tell ✗

Q5.3   Most home cooks don't follow the traditional recipe.

☑ True   ☐ False   ☑ Can't tell ✗

Q5.4   If bacon is used instead of lardons, then garlic should be added to compensate for the dryness.

☐ True   ☐ False   ☑ Can't tell ─

Q5.5   Quiche Lorraine is a vegetarian dish.

☐ True   ☑ False   ☐ Can't tell ✓

Q5.6   Originally, Quiche Lorraine was not a French dish.

☐ True   ☐ False   ☑ Can't tell ✗

Q5.7   The Lorraine region has remained French since it was handed back by Germany in 1918.

☐ True   ☐ False   ☑ Can't tell ✓

Q5.8   Mirabelle liqueur is yellow.

☐ True   ☐ False   ☑ Can't tell ✓

VR 6 Practice	Blu-Ray

TEXT

Blu-Ray – its full name is Blu-Ray Disc (BD) – is the next generation of optical discs developed jointly by a wide range of leading manufacturers, including Dell, Apple, Sony, Philips, Samsung and Sharp. The name of this new technology comes from the fact that it uses a blue-violet laser instead of the red laser currently used by DVD players. Because blue-violet lasers have a shorter wavelength than red lasers, they can be focused with greater precision. This means that data can be packed more tightly onto the disc. Blu-Ray discs can take as much as 25 gigabytes (GB) on each layer. Research carried out by Pioneer has demonstrated that discs can be constructed with up to 20 layers. Hollywood studios have recently announced that they would choose Blu-Ray as their preferred format, and would be releasing titles on both normal DVD and BD format for some time. Although the DVD format will eventually disappear, BD players will be able to play DVDs.

The Blu-Ray Disc Association (BRDA) has indicated that British consumers bought over 400,000 BDs in November 2008, an increase of 165% on October 2008 sales. Such an increase could be reasonably explained by three factors: (i) Blu-Ray has won the format war over DVDs and is bound to become more popular; (ii) The release of popular movies such as Batman on Blu-Ray format just before Christmas has boosted sales; and (iii) as Blu-Ray players become cheaper, BDs will sell more. The BRDA is expecting sales of Blu-Ray players to triple over 2009, reaching 2.5 million units Europe-wide. However, there are strong reasons to suspect that such an increase is unrealistic. No Blu-Ray players are manufactured in the UK and, in the context of a falling Pound and a rising Yen, products manufactured in Japan will become more expensive. BDs also remain comparatively expensive against DVDs and, consequently, the average buyer may delay any purchase until better economic times.

PRACTICE QUESTIONS

7/8 = 87.5%

Q6.1 Everyone should replace their DVD players with a Blu-Ray player as soon as possible as DVDs are being phased out.

☐ True   ☑ False   ☐ Can't tell

Q6.2 Blu-Ray discs are manufactured to store 500GB of data.

☐ True   ☐ False   ☑ Can't tell

Q6.3 Those who purchase Blu-Ray players can discard their DVD players.

☑ True   ☐ False   ☐ Can't tell

Q6.4 Blue-violet lasers are safer than red lasers.

☐ True   ☐ False   ☑ Can't tell

Q6.5 Blu-Ray players would be cheaper if they were manufactured in the UK.

☐ True   ☐ False   ☑ Can't tell

Q6.6 Sales of Blu-Ray players in the UK are expected to increase over 2009.

☑ True   ☐ False   ☐ Can't tell ✗

Q6.7 Batman was not released in DVD format.

☐ True   ☐ False   ☑ Can't tell

Q6.8 Fewer than 200,000 Blu-Ray discs were sold in the UK in October 2008.

☑ True   ☐ False   ☐ Can't tell

VR 7 Practice — Cyanide & Arsenic

TEXT

Cyanide is a substance commonly found in nature, for example in apple pips, apricot stones and coffee beans. Ingested in small amounts it can cause headaches and cardiac palpitations. Cyanide is sometimes described as having a "bitter almond" smell. However, it can sometimes be odourless. In addition, when it does emit a smell, not all humans have the ability to detect it. Death is likely to occur within 5 minutes if as little as 50mg is ingested. More substantial amounts would result in instant death. The poison acts by preventing oxygen from reaching the cells, which quickly affects the heart and the brain. As well as being a well-known poison, cyanide has been used by butterfly collectors – who would crush laurel leaves (which contain cyanide) to produce a preservative liquid – as well as in the gold industry where it is commonly used for mining and electroplating.

Arsenic is also colourless but is totally odourless in its normal state. It is a weak acid which is totally soluble in water. When heated in air at atmospheric pressure, it converts directly from solid form to gaseous form. The fumes from the reaction have a similar smell to garlic. Arsenic was used in Victorian times by women who mixed it with vinegar and chalk and either ingested it or rubbed it into their skin to improve their complexion; the result was a whiter skin which proved that they were not peasants. It has also been abundantly used as a poison, both for humans and also for insects, fungi and bacteria and is often used to preserve wood. Scientists have often exploited its medicinal virtues; originally used for the treatment of syphilis, it has not been superseded in this role by modern antibiotics. It is, however, currently used for the treatment of some leukaemias, and psoriasis, and new research suggests that it may be better than iodine-124 in locating tumours when doing PET-scan imaging.

PRACTICE QUESTIONS

Q7.1 Most humans would detect cyanide's bitter almond smell when it is present.

  ☐ True   ☐ False   ☐ Can't tell

Q7.2 Butterflies caught by collectors were killed using a cyanide-based solution made from laurel leaves.

  ☐ True   ☐ False   ☐ Can't tell

Q7.3 Humans should avoid consuming large quantities of apples, apricots and coffee.

  ☐ True   ☐ False   ☐ Can't tell

Q7.4 Cyanide is a by-product of gold mining.

  ☐ True   ☐ False   ☐ Can't tell

Q7.5 Arsenic does not exist in liquid form.

  ☐ True   ☐ False   ☐ Can't tell

Q7.6 Iodine-124 is currently being used to locate tumours.

  ☐ True   ☐ False   ☐ Can't tell

Q7.7 Arsenic and cyanide are both toxic to insects.

  ☐ True   ☐ False   ☐ Can't tell

Q7.8 Someone who was being poisoned by ingesting water containing arsenic would not be able to detect its presence.

  ☐ True   ☐ False   ☐ Can't tell

VR 8
Practice
Chocolate

TEXT

It has often been said that chocolate contains caffeine but this is a myth. In fact, cocoa contains a substance called theobromine, which is a stimulant that is found only in cocoa. Caffeine may be artificially added by chocolate-makers but is not present naturally. Both substances are cardiovascular stimulants. However, fundamentally the effects of theobromine differ widely from those of caffeine. Whilst caffeine is physically addictive, increases emotional stress, stimulates the respiratory system and increases alertness, theobromine is not addictive, is a mild antidepressant, stimulates the muscular system and increases the feeling of well-being. Smoking cigarettes accelerates the dissipation of both substances from the system. As for tea, although it contains more caffeine than coffee, a typical serving contains much less, as tea is normally brewed much weaker.

As well as theobromine, chocolate contains other compounds which are each credited with a range of benefits; for example, recent studies have concluded that chocolate can reduce cholesterol levels through the polyphenols that it naturally contains. Consequently, some manufacturers have sought to fully exploit these newly found health benefits in their advertising and others are going even further by introducing new ingredients into their chocolate products to provide consumers with further benefits. We are now seeing calcium-enriched chocolates which strengthen bones, and can prevent dental caries, osteoporosis and even colon cancer. Soy fibre is being introduced into chocolate to help with cholesterol reduction and phytostanols (saturated phytosterols such as sitostanol and campestanol) are currently being studied as potential cholesterol-lowering compounds for incorporation into chocolate. Soy fibre is derived from the soya bean. Due to its neutral taste and light colour, soy fibre can be incorporated into a variety of high-fibre and reduced-calorie products without affecting traditional quality. A particularly new area of development is the addition of mood-enhancing plants or compounds such as ginseng, ginko or even royal jelly. This has led to the introduction of a wide range of chocolates which claim to improve brain activity, enhance memory or even have an aphrodisiac effect.

PRACTICE QUESTIONS

Q8.1 Drinking tea may lead to increased emotional stress.

☐ True ☐ False ☐ Can't tell

Q8.2 Smoking compensates for the effects of caffeine and theobromine.

☐ True ☐ False ☐ Can't tell

Q8.3 Chocolate is not addictive.

☐ True ☐ False ☐ Can't tell

Q8.4 Chocolate can only contain caffeine if coffee is mixed with it.

☐ True ☐ False ☐ Can't tell

Q8.5 Phytostanols are substances occurring naturally in plants.

☐ True ☐ False ☐ Can't tell

Q8.6 Soy fibre contains phytostanols.

☐ True ☐ False ☐ Can't tell

Q8.7 The risks of developing osteoporosis can be reduced by eating calcium-enriched foods.

☐ True ☐ False ☐ Can't tell

Q8.8 Some of the advertised health benefits of enhanced chocolate are unproven.

☐ True ☐ False ☐ Can't tell

VR 9
Practice
Pregnancy Food

TEXT

Pregnant women should be aware of the consequence of eating cheese during pregnancy. Cheese constitutes an important source of calcium and protein to pregnant women; however, some varieties of cheese may encourage the growth of bacteria which could harm an unborn child. Women avoiding high-risk cheese are very unlikely to be affected by such bacteria such as listeria. Hard cheeses such as Cheddar, Edam, Gruyère, feta and Parmesan, and soft and processed cheeses such as Boursin, goat cheese without a white rind, mozzarella and ricotta are safe to eat in pregnancy because listeria is present in such small numbers that the risk is considered extremely small. Mould-ripened soft cheeses such as Brie and Camembert, blue-veined cheeses such as Roquefort and Stilton, and soft unpasteurised cheeses must be avoided. All yoghurts, crème fraiche and sour cream are safe to eat, whether they are natural, flavoured or biologically active.

Fish is a good meal choice during pregnancy as it contains omega-3 fatty acids that help baby's brain development. However, the expectant mother should avoid some varieties such as shark and swordfish, which contain high levels of methyl-mercury, a substance which may affect baby's nervous system. These fish live longer and are therefore accumulating more mercury in their flesh than other fish. Be aware too that most types of fish contain traces of mercury, so a pregnant woman may want to limit her weekly consumption of safer varieties too. It is recommended that no more than 350g of lower-mercury fish such as salmon, shrimp or canned light tuna be consumed in a week (which is equivalent to approximately two meals). Of those 350g, only half should come from canned "white" albacore tuna, which tends to contain more mercury than light tuna (which is a mix of different low-mercury tuna species). Women who have any doubt about mercury levels or the provenance of the fish should limit their fish consumption to 175g per week.

PRACTICE QUESTIONS

Q9.1 Pregnant women should avoid goat cheese with a white rind.

☐ True   ☐ False   ☐ Can't tell

Q9.2 A pregnant woman eating no other cheese than Cheddar cannot get listeria infection.

☐ True   ☐ False   ☐ Can't tell

Q9.3 Pregnant women should steer clear of cheese.

☐ True   ☐ False   ☐ Can't tell

Q9.4 A sandwich made only from ham and Gruyère between two slices of bread is safe for a pregnant woman to eat.

☐ True   ☐ False   ☐ Can't tell

Q9.5 It would normally be considered safe for a pregnant woman to eat 150g of a fish pie made exclusively of the following ingredients: salmon, white albacore tuna, shrimp, crème fraiche, Cheddar, Parmesan.

☐ True   ☐ False   ☐ Can't tell

Q9.6 White tuna is the species of tuna with the longest life expectancy.

☐ True   ☐ False   ☐ Can't tell

Q9.7 Once ingested by a fish, methyl-mercury tends to stay in its body for some time.

☐ True   ☐ False   ☐ Can't tell

Q9.8 Assuming all other factors equal, a young fish from one species will contain less mercury than an older fish from the same species.

☐ True   ☐ False   ☐ Can't tell

| VR 10 Practice | The Grass is Greener |

TEXT – LETTER DATED 5 JANUARY

Dear Sir

I am writing regarding the parking ticket which I found on my car this morning and would like to explain why I believe it should be cancelled. On 16 December, I parked my car legally within the white markings on Green Avenue, a small street parallel to the street in which I live. This is a road where anyone is free to park for free all year round. This morning, as I was setting out for work, I found my car on a nearby piece of grass, with a parking ticket for £120, stating that I was being fined because my car was illegally parked on the grass. This is NOT where I had left it.

I gather from a notice that I found on a lamp post near where I originally parked the car that the road has been resurfaced recently. The notice was dated 17 December and announced that parking would be suspended between 19 December and 24 December, both dates included, to allow resurfacing work to take place during that time. It was confirmed to me by the Council that the resurfacing work did indeed take place at some stage between those two dates. Because I was away from the country between 18 December and 2 January, I was not able to move my car from its normal parking space and I know from having talked to neighbours that the workers moved the car before starting the resurfacing work. Since I was not responsible for moving the car, I don't see why I should have to pay for it!

I feel that this parking fine is unfair because the notice given to remove my car was posted after I had parked it there and did not give me enough time to remove the car. It is also unfair of you to expect that, around Christmas time, people would be around to read the notice in the first place.

I therefore hope that you will cancel the ticket and look forward to hearing from you soon with the good news.

Best regards
John Rover

PRACTICE QUESTIONS

Q10.1 The car's owner was fined for being in breach of the parking suspension.

☐ True ☐ False ☐ Can't tell

Q10.2 The car remained parked on the grass for at least a week.

☐ True ☐ False ☐ Can't tell

Q10.3 John Rover lives in a street where parking is normally free.

☐ True ☐ False ☐ Can't tell

Q10.4 The resurfacing work lasted 5 days.

☐ True ☐ False ☐ Can't tell

Q10.5 John Rover did not use his car on 17 December.

☐ True ☐ False ☐ Can't tell

Q10.6 Although dated 17 December, the parking suspension notice was
not placed on the lamp post before 18 December.

☐ True ☐ False ☐ Can't tell

Q10.7 The parking ticket was placed on the car on or before 24 December.

☐ True ☐ False ☐ Can't tell

Q10.8 Legally, councils are only required to give two days' notice for
parking suspensions.

☐ True ☐ False ☐ Can't tell

VR 11
Practice
The Bard

TEXT

After three years of meticulous research, X-rays and infrared imaging, experts have finally lifted all doubts: the only known portrait of William Shakespeare painted whilst he was alive has been found! The painting was unveiled on Monday in London by Professor Stanley Wells, president of the Foundation Shakespeare Birthplace, an association which manages the museum in Stratford-upon-Avon, where the poet was born.

The painting was made in 1610, several years before the death of the great English poet and writer. It is part of a collection owned for centuries by the family of Alex Cobbe, a restorer of objects of art who inherited it. The painting was very well appreciated within his family but no one had made the link with the poet until Alex saw a portrait of Shakespeare with an uncanny similarity to his own painting at the National Portrait Gallery in London. This was a painting from the Folger Shakespeare Library in Washington, and which had, for a long time, been deemed to have been painted whilst Shakespeare was still alive, before analyses made 70 years ago concluded that the paint dated from the 19th century.

Realising that he was the owner of the original version, which had been copied, he contacted Professor Stanley Wells who was at first dubious because the oldest known paintings and busts of Shakespeare had, until then, all been done just after his death in 1616.

Professor Rupert Featherstone of the University of Cambridge looked at the pigments used whilst experts from the University of Hamburg dated the oak plank on which the portrait was painted. Their conclusions were positive: the painting was made when Shakespeare was still alive. Another favourable point: the painting was found by the Cobbes with another portrait which represented the Count of Southampton, one of Shakespeare's main financial sponsors.

PRACTICE QUESTIONS

Q11.1 The Cobbes' painting was made approximately six years before Shakespeare's death.

☐ True ☐ False ☐ Can't tell

Q11.2 The Cobbes' painting was the only portrait of Shakespeare ever painted during his lifetime.

☐ True ☐ False ☐ Can't tell

Q11.3 The Folger Shakespeare Library copy of the painting was painted 70 years ago.

☐ True ☐ False ☐ Can't tell

Q11.4 Shakespeare was born in a museum.

☐ True ☐ False ☐ Can't tell

Q11.5 The portrait was painted on wood rather than on a canvas.

☐ True ☐ False ☐ Can't tell

Q11.6 The Count of Southampton met Shakespeare during his lifetime.

☐ True ☐ False ☐ Can't tell

Q11.7 The Folger Shakespeare Library copy of the painting was made over three centuries after the original portrait was painted.

☐ True ☐ False ☐ Can't tell

Q11.8 Alex Cobbe restored the original Shakespeare portrait inherited by his family.

☐ True ☐ False ☐ Can't tell

VR 12 Practice — Delay Compensation Package

TEXT

Euro MPs have recently adopted a new law compensating bus, coach and boat passengers for delays and cancellations.

Maritime transport companies will have the obligation to "provide information to their passengers as well as compensation if their journey is disrupted or interrupted", the Parliament explains. Compensation will vary between 25% of the price of the ticket for delays between one and two hours and 50% if the delay exceeds two hours. Compensation is 100% of the ticket price if the company does not provide suitable alternative means of transport or information on alternative means of transport.

For buses and coaches, companies will also need to provide a substitute or information about substitute modes of transport. If required, they will also need to pay half the ticket price.

New EU legislation had already been adopted in 2005 for plane delays, with passengers denied boarding because of overbooking, or delays caused by other airline hiccups, receiving compensation of 250 Euros for short-haul flights, rising to 600 Euros for long-haul flights. If a flight is cancelled, airlines have to give passengers meals, refreshments and overnight accommodation (including a transfer to the hotel) free of charge or find them alternative transport to their final destination. Passengers are also entitled to complimentary refreshments on board the aircraft if they are delayed beyond a specified number of hours, which depends on the distance they are due to fly. Those who are most affected are the budget airlines, as the compensation sums represent a huge proportion of their average fares.

PRACTICE QUESTIONS

Q12.1 A delay of 1 hour on the bus will give rise to compensation of 25% of the price of the ticket.

☐ True   ☐ False   ☐ Can't tell

Q12.2 Compensation in the airline industry is not related to the cost of the ticket.

☐ True   ☐ False   ☐ Can't tell

Q12.3 Compensation for airline delays cannot exceed 600 Euros.

☐ True   ☐ False   ☐ Can't tell

Q12.4 The introduction of the new compensation rules will lead to an increase in ticket prices.

☐ True   ☐ False   ☐ Can't tell

Q12.5 It is possible for airline delay compensation to be higher than the price paid for the ticket.

☐ True   ☐ False   ☐ Can't tell

Q12.6 It is possible for ferry delay compensation to be higher than the price paid for the ticket.

☐ True   ☐ False   ☐ Can't tell

Q12.7 Boat companies are legally obliged to organise an alternative mode of transport for their passengers.

☐ True   ☐ False   ☐ Can't tell

Q12.8 All airline passengers who are entitled to the 600 Euro compensation package for long-haul flights are also entitled to complimentary refreshments on board the aircraft.

☐ True   ☐ False   ☐ Can't tell

11 Verbal Reasoning Answers to Practice Questions

VR 1 – FINANCIAL CRISIS

Q1.1 – CAN'T TELL
All we know is that the merger followed the collapse of Lehman Brothers. Although there might have been a link, the text does not suggest any.

Q1.2 – TRUE
The text clearly states that American banks sold the sub-prime debt to banks around the world and that it was the failure to repay those sub-prime debts which started the collapse.

Q1.3 – CAN'T TELL
It is commonly accepted that bankers' greed played a key role in the onset of the financial crisis; however, for the purpose of the exam, you must stick to what the text is saying. The text states that "some commentators have said that bankers' greed was a contributor to the problem". It does not specify the extent of the role played by greed, or imply whether the financial crisis could have avoided been avoided if greed had not been present. We simply know that it contributed.

Q1.4 – TRUE
The second sentence of the text explicitly states that the source of the crisis is linked to US banks. Again, there might have been other reasons elsewhere, but you must stick to what the text says and not use any additional knowledge or preconceptions you may have.

Q1.5 – CAN'T TELL
At the very end, the text says that pyramid schemes are illegal in the UK, which is not the same as saying that they do not exist. The text contains no information to suggest that any pyramid schemes actually operate in the UK. It is highly likely that several are in existence, and you may well be aware of some of them; however, you must ensure that you do not use any external knowledge to answer the question. Based on what we are given, we cannot say whether pyramid schemes exist in the UK.

Q1.6 – FALSE
There are several elements in the text which point towards a "False" answer. First, the beginning of the second paragraph implies that the alleged fraud was in addition to the financial crisis. Second, the second paragraph clearly indicates that the alleged fraud affected rich individuals, whereas the first paragraph is clear in saying that the financial crisis had its roots in the "less well-off" population. Although it is possible that the alleged fraud contributed to some extent to the financial crisis, the text does not allow us to say that it was a key trigger.

Q1.7 – CAN'T TELL
The text talks about a $50bn fraud. We do not know whether this was the total amount of money invested by those who participated in the scheme or whether this was the amount of money that the financier made. In addition, we are told that this is an "alleged" fraud, which places further ambiguity on the statement.

Q1.8 – TRUE
The text clearly states that pyramid schemes are unsustainable.

VR 2 – GLOBAL WARMING

Q2.1 – TRUE
The text suggests that there are different schools of thought on the topic of global warming; however those who criticise these measures argue that they will have little effect, not that they will have no effect at all. It is possible that such effect is very minimal (it is impossible from the text to determine how much of an effect this is likely to have), but this is enough to answer "true" to this question.

Q2.2 – FALSE
The text merely states that they believe it will have little effect. This is not the same as saying that there is no need to take action.

Q2.3 – CAN'T TELL
The text says that China is one of the biggest contributors. There is no suggestion that it is the biggest contributor of carbon emissions.

Q2.4 – CAN'T TELL
Nothing in the text suggests that global warming is used as an excuse to reduce the number of cars (which does not mean that it isn't the case).

Q2.5 – CAN'T TELL
The text states that the average sea level will rise by between 18 and 59cm. Since this is the average sea level, this means that some sea levels are expected to rise by less than 18cm and others by more than 59cm. In fact the previous sentence says that individual sea levels could rise by anything between 9cm and 88cm. This may or may not include Britain; nothing in the text points one way or another.

Q2.6 – TRUE
The text states "a reduction of the ice cap in the northern hemisphere, whereas in Antarctica (i.e. in the southern hemisphere) the melting of the ice cap would be more than offset by heavier snow falls, with the snow then freezing over the existing layer of ice".

The use of the word "whereas" opposes two statements with the events in Antarctica being opposed to the events in the northern hemisphere. Since the northern hemisphere ice cap is reducing, this implies that the Antarctica ice cap is not (though this does not necessarily mean that it is actually increasing; it could simply be remaining stable). However, the phrase "more than offset" indicates that snow will be falling at a higher rate than the ice is melting, which points towards an actual increase of the ice cap.

Q2.7 – CAN'T TELL
The text does mention at the end that some areas of the world may see some benefits but there is nothing about these countries not experiencing any negative impacts. This lack of information means that we cannot conclude decisively.

Q2.8 – TRUE
We are told that the average world temperature will rise by between 1.4 and 5.8 °C. So, it is possible that the average rise will be 5.8 °C. This then means that some countries will see rises below 5.8 and some countries will see rises above 5.8. The use of the word "may" in the assertion makes it a true statement according to the text. If the assertion had been "some countries will experience a rise of temperature of over 5.8 °C", then we could not have concluded either way since we cannot know for sure what the average rise will be and therefore whether any countries will actually experience such a high rise.

VR 3 – FREE MUSEUM ENTRY

Q3.1 – FALSE
The text states that some of the increase is due to the same people visiting museums more often. This suggests there are other reasons. There

Q3.2 – TRUE
On average the increase was 70%. Since we know that at least one museum had an increase of 111% then there has to be others with less than 70% increase in visitors.

Q3.3 – FALSE
The text states that the subsidies are mostly directed towards London museums. The use of the term "mostly" implies that others have benefited too, though perhaps not to the same extent. It is therefore incorrect that only London museums have benefited.

Q3.4 – CAN'T TELL
The question uses the word "solely". It could only be true if the text clearly showed that there could be no other explanation for the increased visitor numbers than the introduction of the new policy. The text states that the number of visitors increased the following year but does not say why. It also suggests a link with the fact that some museums have refurbished their facilities, so this may have accounted for some of the increase. For statement Q3.4 to be false, we would need proof that there was at least another factor which contributed to the increased visitor numbers. We know that there is a possible link with the refurbishment and new facilities of some museums but we don't know whether this actually had an impact. We therefore cannot conclude either way.

This is a typical case of a question where you have to leave your common sense on the side and solely concentrate on what the text is telling you. To most people, it is obvious that the new policy cannot be the sole contributor to the increased visitor number and that, consequently, the statement in Q3.4 is actually false. However, the text is inconclusive in that regard. It only suggests that there may be a link with some other factors.

Q3.5 – FALSE
The first sentence says that "In 2001, the government reintroduced free entry into museums ...", which means that it had been done before.

Q3.6 – CAN'T TELL
The figure of £2.21 billion – £1.68 billion = £0.53 billion = £530 million over 3 years is correct. However, all we know is that this is what the Chancellor promised. We cannot say when this <u>will</u> actually happen.

Q3.7 – CAN'T TELL
We know that the free-entry policy will be extended by at least 3 years. The text therefore leaves open the possibility that it may be extended by more. The last sentence indicates that the Arts may suffer from the current financial crisis and the Olympic Games, but there is no indication that this will affect the free-entry policy. There is no indication either that it will not be affected; therefore we cannot conclude either way.

Q3.8 – CAN'T TELL
What the second paragraph tells us is that independent museums have seen a decline since the introduction of free entry. Therefore a fee-paying policy would be fairer to <u>independent</u> museums because it would place them on an even footing. We are being asked to determine whether a fee-paying entry policy would be fairer to <u>smaller</u> museums. This would be true if the text showed that the independent museums are also the smaller ones. Unfortunately, the text does not allow us to determine this; therefore we cannot conclude either way.

VR 4 – EEC, EU, EURO

Q4.1 – FALSE
The Eurozone is defined as the 15 countries from the EU who have adopted the Euro. The text says that, in addition, 11 non-EU countries have adopted the Euro including Monaco. Therefore Monaco, although it uses the Euro, is not in the officially-defined Eurozone.

Q4.2 – CAN'T TELL
Although, if you know your history, you will know that this statement is true, we cannot conclude it from the text. The text tells us that in 1993, the statement was true. For the statement to be true currently, we would need confirmation that none of the original countries have left the EU since 1993. The text does not say anything on the matter. It only states that there are now 27 countries but does not list them. Remember to base your conclusions on the text only and not on your general knowledge.

Q4.3 – FALSE

The first paragraph does state that the <u>main</u> EU institutions are in Belgium and France. However, there are other institutions which reside some-where else; in fact the text states that the European Central Bank is in Germany. The statement that all institutions are based in Belgium or in France is therefore false.

Q4.4 – FALSE

We know that both countries have declined to join the Euro, but that is not an indication of future intention. The first sentence of the second para-graph says that the UK has adopted a wait-and-see policy, which means that it remains open. Therefore the fact that neither countries intend to adopt the Euro is incorrect.

Q4.5 – TRUE

The second paragraph states clearly that interest rates would be set by the European Central Bank in Frankfurt. It also later states that if the UK had joined the Euro, the Bank of England would not have been able to reduce interest rates drastically to boost the UK economy.

Q4.6 – CAN'T TELL

The only mention of the US is in a statement which says that "It has long been argued that the UK economy is more in line with US economy than with European economy and that therefore it needs to keep closer links with US interest rates than European interest rates." There is nothing in the text which suggests that, if two countries have economies which are aligned, they would benefit overall by having a common currency (since the text presents both pros and cons). This is all speculative and nothing in the text allows us to draw such a definitive conclusion.

Q4.7 – CAN'T TELL

The text says that the EU includes 27 independent sovereign countries, but this does not mean that there are not any other independent sovereign countries outside the EU. The fact that Andorra is a non-EU country (which the text states) does not mean that it is not an independent sover-eign country. In the absence of any further information, we cannot con-clude either way.

Q4.8 – CAN'T TELL

What the text says is that, should the UK adopt the Euro, UK interest rates would be set by the European Central Bank in Frankfurt. There is no mention of the Bank of England disappearing (e.g. to fulfil other roles). However, since there is no mention of the Bank of England remaining either, we cannot conclude either way.

VR 5 – COQ AU VIN & QUICHE LORRAINE

Q5.1 – FALSE
The list of main ingredients in the first sentence does not contain bacon. Bacon may be used as a substitute for lardons and therefore cannot be labelled "essential".

Q5.2 – TRUE
The second paragraph is clear in suggesting that thick bacon can be used as a substitute for lardons.

Q5.3 – TRUE
The traditional recipe uses rooster. The first paragraph states that most home cooks use chicken as a substitute. Therefore, it follows that most home cooks don't follow the traditional recipe.

Q5.4 – CAN'T TELL
The text says that using bacon makes the dish drier. The text also says that occasionally garlic is used. What we don't know is what the effect of garlic is. Although there does not seem to be much logic behind the statement, we cannot actually say whether there is a link between the two.

Q5.5 – FALSE
We are told that Quiche Lorraine is made with lardons. The first paragraph clearly states that lardons are made of pork, so Quiche Lorraine contains meat.

Q5.6 – TRUE
Quiche Lorraine comes from the Lorraine region, which, the text states, was first taken by France in 1648 (i.e. the 17th century). The first sentence of the second paragraph says that the dish dates back to the 16th century, i.e. before it became French.

Q5.7 – CAN'T TELL
The text does not state what happened to the Lorraine region after 1918 and does not state anywhere that it has remained French since then (Note: in fact it briefly became German again during WWII, but this is not

information which can be found in the text). Therefore we cannot conclude either way.

Q5.8 – CAN'T TELL
The Mirabelle fruit is yellow, but there is no indication of the colour of the liqueur.

VR 6 – BLU-RAY

Q6.1 – FALSE
If the industry wanted people to switch to BD players as soon as possible then they would only release new titles in BD format (since BD readers can also read DVDs). The fact that titles will still be released in DVD format for some time means that there is no rush to switch to BD.

Q6.2 – CAN'T TELL
We know that each disc layer can take 25 GB and we know that Pioneer has "demonstrated that Blu-ray discs can be constructed with up to 20 layers. Therefore, 20 x 25 = 500MB is the total possible capacity of a Blu-ray disc; however, we can't tell whether they are or will be actually manufactured at maximum capacity. We simply know that it possible to achieve this level.

Q6.3 – TRUE
Those who purchase BD players will also be able to play DVDs on them. Therefore DVD players will become redundant and can therefore be discarded.

Q6.4 – CAN'T TELL
The text does not deal with the safety aspect of the two types of lasers. Therefore we simply cannot answer the question.

Q6.5 – CAN'T TELL
What the text actually says is that because Blu-Ray readers are manufactured abroad, the fluctuations in exchange rates will make them more expensive than what they cost at present, i.e. we are comparing the cost to a UK consumer of a foreign product before and after currency fluctuation. There is nothing to indicate whether manufacturing the product in the UK would be cheaper. For example, if we assume that the current cost of a Blu-Ray player is £1,000, then exchange rate pressures may increase this cost to £1,200, say. But this may still be cheap in comparison to what it

would cost to manufacture the product in the UK (which could be £2,000 say).

Q6.6 – CAN'T TELL
We know that sales of Blu-Ray readers are expected to triple over 2009, but that this figure is Europe-wide. We are not told of expectations over the UK. All we know about the UK is that the sales of Blu-Ray discs has increased (which does not necessarily mean that the sales of readers has increased and, in any case, a past increase in sales does not necessarily translate into a future increase in sales). So, although there may be good reasons to believe that the statement is true, we cannot conclude for certain on the basis of the text. In fact, the final sentence suggests that economic uncertainty and adverse exchange rates could go against Blu-Ray in the short term.

Q6.7 – CAN'T TELL
We are told that Batman was released in Blu-Ray format but nothing indicates that it wasn't released in DVD format as well. Therefore we cannot tell either way.

Q6.8 – TRUE
The sale of 400,000 discs in November 2008 represents an increase of 165% on October 2008 figures. Therefore the number of discs sold in October would be calculated as 400,000 / 2.65, which is below 200,000.

VR7 – CYANIDE & ARSENIC

Q7.1 – CAN'T TELL
We know that some humans cannot detect its smell; however, we don't know the percentage of humans who can. Therefore we cannot say whether "most humans" (i.e. over 50%) would detect the smell when present.

Q7.2 – CAN'T TELL
The text says the cyanide in the crushed leaves was used to make a preservative liquid. However, we don't know how the butterflies were killed.

Q7.3 – CAN'T TELL
We are not told how much fruit a human being would need to eat to suffer harmful effects and whether anyone could realistically eat all of these in a reasonable amount of time for the cyanide concentration to be harmful.

There is certainly nothing in the text which suggests that eating too much of the cyanide-containing fruit could be detrimental to humans. We therefore simply cannot conclude whether the statement is true or false from the information given.

Q7.4 – CAN'T TELL
The text only says that cyanide is used in mining. We can't conclude whether cyanide is a by-product of mining or not.

Q7.5 – CAN'T TELL
We are told that arsenic converts directly from solid to gaseous form when heated in air at atmospheric pressure. Nothing indicates that a liquid form is not possible under different conditions.

Q7.6 – CAN'T TELL
We are told that arsenic is better than iodine-124 to locate tumours; however, we don't know whether iodine-124 is what is being used currently.

Q7.7 – CAN'T TELL
We are told explicitly that arsenic is a poison to insects, so the answer now depends on whether cyanide is toxic to insects or not. Although we know from the text that cyanide is toxic to humans and that it is also being used in a preservative liquid for butterflies; we cannot conclude that it is toxic to insects.

Q7.8 – CAN'T TELL
Several elements point towards this statement being true including the following: (i) arsenic is totally soluble in water; (ii) arsenic is colourless; and (iii) arsenic is odourless in its normal state. However, the text does not say anything about taste.

VR8 – CHOCOLATE

Q8.1 – TRUE
From the text, we know that tea contains caffeine and that caffeine increases emotional stress. Therefore we can conclude that drinking tea (and the caffeine within it) may lead to increased emotional stress. If the statement had said that "drinking tea always leads to increased to emotional stress" then the answer would have been "Can't tell". Indeed the text tells us that it is caffeine (and not tea) which leads to increased emotional stress. It could well be that there are other substances in tea which

counteract the effects of caffeine. We simply don't know. What makes this statement true is the presence of the word "may" within it, which simply indicates that it is possible, rather than definite.

Q8.2 – CAN'T TELL
The text says that smoking cigarettes accelerates the dissipation of both substances from the system. This is not the same as compensating for the effects. Nothing in the text mentions the impact of cigarette smoking on the effect of caffeine.

Q8.3 – CAN'T TELL
From the text, we know that theobromine is not addictive, but that does not mean that chocolate isn't.

Q8.4 – FALSE
The text tells us that chocolate does not contain caffeine naturally and that any caffeine found in chocolate has been added artificially. However, this could be achieved by other means than by adding coffee (for example, the text tells us that there is caffeine in tea).

Q8.5 – CAN'T TELL
The name "phytostanols" contains the root "phyton" which, in Greek, does mean "plant" and the context does suggest that phytostanols may be a natural substance; however, the text itself (remember: all that matters is what we can conclude from the text itself) does not give enough information to enable us to conclude that this is the case.

Q8.6 – CAN'T TELL
Soy fibre and phytostanols are both discussed within the text, one as a cholesterol-lowering tool and the other one simply as being under investigation. There is nothing to suggest whether soy fibre contains phytostanols.

Q8.7 – TRUE
The text states that calcium-enriched chocolates can prevent osteoporosis. This suggests that it is either the calcium, the chocolate or both which prevent osteoporosis. However, the context here is a discussion on how different types of new ingredients can bring different health benefits, so clearly we are being told that it is the calcium enrichment which is making a difference and we can generalise the statement.

Q8.8 – CAN'T TELL
The text presents some benefits as proven (e.g. soy fibre lowering choles-terol, calcium enrichment strengthening bones, preventing dental caries, etc.) but also says that some of the benefits are just claims made by manufacturers (e.g. improving brain activity, enhancing memory, aphrodi-siac). The use of the word "claim" suggests that the author may have a cynical view of such claims; however it does not mean that they are un-proven (indeed, it could simply be due to the author's ignorance of such proofs). The only thing that we know is not proven is the cholesterol-reducing effect of phytostanols, but, as far as we know from the text, no manufacturer has made such a claim.

VR9 – PREGNANCY FOOD

Q9.1 – CAN'T TELL
We know that goat cheese without a white rind is safe. However, we don't know if the presence of a white rind makes it unsafe.

Q9.2 – FALSE
The text states that Cheddar is safe to eat, but then goes on to explain that this is because the level of bacteria is so low that the risk is extremely small. In addition, the final sentence of the first paragraph states that women avoiding high-risk cheese are very unlikely to be affected by lis-teria. Although the risk is very small, it still exists and it is therefore incor-rect to state that a woman eating Cheddar only cannot get listeria infec-tion. If the wording of the statement were "is unlikely to get listeria infec-tion", the statement would be true.

Q9.3 – FALSE
The recommendations are that many cheeses are actually on the whole, safe for pregnant women. The first paragraph also states that cheese can be beneficial to pregnant women. The text actually encourages pregnant women to eat cheese, though remaining careful about which they should eat. Nowhere does it state that women should steer clear of cheese, even if it reminds the reader that every cheese has its risk.

Q9.4 – CAN'T TELL
We know that Gruyere is safe, but we don't know whether ham and bread are safe.

Q9.5 – TRUE
The whole meal weighs 150g so, although we don't know exactly how much fish it contains, we know it will be under the 175g which constitutes the absolute safe limit for women who have doubts. All the ingredients described are either safe cheeses or low-mercury fish and we know there are no other ingredients ("made exclusively of the following ingredients") so the pie is safe to eat in this quantity.

Q9.6 – CAN'T TELL
All we know from the text is that (i) longer living fish tend to have greater mercury levels and that (ii) canned white tuna contains more mercury than light tuna, which is a mix of low-mercury tuna species. We know nothing about other species of tuna (which are not being canned) and therefore cannot conclude either way.

Q9.7 – TRUE
This is the principle which underlines the whole of the second paragraph. We are being told that fish which live longer are accumulating more mercury (hence why they may be unsafe). The word "accumulating" is an explicit answer to the question.

Q9.8 – TRUE
We know from the text that mercury builds up in the body with age. Therefore it makes sense for a young fish to have less mercury than an older fish of the same species. However, there is always a risk that external conditions such as living in a mercury-polluted river or sea could make this assumption wrong. But since the question says that we must assume that all other factors are equal, then we can confidently conclude that the assertion is true.

VR10 – THE GRASS IS GREENER

Q10.1 – FALSE
The parking suspension applies to the bay in the street in which he normally parks. Because John Rover left his car in that bay before the resurfacing took place, the car was moved onto a piece of grass and he was fined for parking on the grass (as the ticket says) and not for remaining parked in the bay after the suspension took effect (although he was also guilty of that latter offence, this is not what he was fined for).

Q10.2 – TRUE
We know that the letter was dated 5 January, on which date he discovered the car parked on the grass, together with the ticket.

We also know that the car was moved before the resurfacing commenced (from the neighbour's testimony) and that the resurfacing work took place between 19 and 24 December. This means that the car was moved before 24 December. So the car was on the grass at least between 24 December and 5 January, which is over a week.

Q10.3 – CAN'T TELL
All we know is that parking is normally free on Green Avenue, which is parallel to the street in which he lives. We don't know whether parking is free in his own street.

Q10.4 – CAN'T TELL
We know that parking was suspended between 19 December and 24 December (i.e. 6 days) and that, during that time, the road was resurfaced. We don't know whether the resurfacing took place during the entire period or not.

Q10.5 – CAN'T TELL
We know that he used his car on 16 December since he said he parked it in Green Avenue on that day and that he left the country on 18 December. There is nothing in the text which enables us to conclude that he did not use his car on 17 December.

Q10.6 – CAN'T TELL
All we know is that he did not see the notice on 17 December. We cannot conclude it wasn't there (though it is possible).

Q10.7 – CAN'T TELL
The parking ticket was placed on the car because the car was parked on the grass. The car would have been moved onto the grass between the time the notice was put up and the time the work started. So this could be at any time between 17 December and 24 December.

However, we don't know when the ticket was placed on the car. This could have been at any time before 5 January when John Rover found it on his car.

Q10.8 – CAN'T TELL
The text does not deal with the legal aspect. All we know is that the notice was signed two days before the day of the suspension. Whether this was legal or not cannot be concluded from the text as it stands.

VR11 – THE BARD

Q11.1 – TRUE
We are told that the painting was made in 1610, several years before his death. Later on, we are told he died in 1616. Since we ignore in which month he died or the painting was made, we can conclude that the use of the word "approximately" makes the sentence true.

Q11.2 – CAN'T TELL
We know that it was painted during his lifetime and that all other known pieces were done afterwards. But we cannot conclude definitively that there are no other paintings which were also done during his lifetime. Some may well be hidden in other places. This is reiterated in the first paragraph which states that it is the "only *known* portrait".

Q11.3 – FALSE
It was found to be a fake 70 years ago but it was painted in the 19th century, therefore over 100 years ago.

Q11.4 – CAN'T TELL
Although this seems absurd, we can't actually conclude either way from the text. The text says: "Foundation Shakespeare Birthplace, an association which manages the museum in Stratford-upon-Avon, where the poet was born." What this really says is that Shakespeare was born in Stratford-upon-Avon rather than in the museum, but, since we don't actually know where exactly he was born in that town, we can't conclude that he wasn't born in a museum.

Q11.5 – TRUE
The text states that the portrait was painted on an oak plank.

Q11.6 – CAN'T TELL
We know that he lived at the same time as he was financing him, but nothing in the text links the two men as having met. We only know their two portraits were found in the same place.

Q11.7 – FALSE
The painting was made in 1610. The copy dates from the 19th century, i.e. between 1800 and 1899, which makes it between 190 and 289 years later i.e. under three centuries.

Q11.8 – CAN'T TELL
We know that he owns the painting and is a restorer, but we don't know whether he actually restored the portrait.

VR12 – DELAY COMPENSATION PACKAGE

Q12.1 – CAN'T TELL
The text is actually ambiguous on this matter. Intuitively one would think that buses and coaches would follow the same rules as boats, but the text only mentions the need to pay half of the ticket price "if required" without mentioning anything about how such requirement is assessed or whether the 25% also applies for smaller delays.

Q12.2 – TRUE
The amounts are fixed and therefore are not linked to ticket prices.

Q12.3 – FALSE
As well as the potential maximum of 600 Euros, the text also mentions having to provide free accommodation, meals, etc. This will add to the costs.

Q12.4 – CAN'T TELL
Although this is a possibility, there is nothing in the text that remotely addresses this issue.

Q12.5 – TRUE
Since the compensation amount is fixed at an arbitrary level, it is of course possible that an airline with cheap tickets could pay more in compensation than the price paid for the ticket. This is a fact that is emphasised in the last sentence of the text.

Q12.6 – FALSE
There is no mention in the text of any reason why compensation should go over 100%. In fact, we know that it would normally be 50% and would only increase to 100% if no information was provided.

Q12.7 – FALSE

Companies only have an obligation to provide information. We can get this from two places: the first sentence of the second paragraph states this explicitly; also, the compensation of 100% is only payable if companies fail to provide alternative means of transport or information on alternative modes of transport. There is therefore no need for them to actually organise it.

Q12.8 – CAN'T TELL

The 600 Euros are payable for delays but we don't know how many hours of delay are needed. We also know that there are complimentary drinks on board the aircraft for those who have been delayed beyond a specified number of hours, though the text says nothing about what those hours are. Therefore we have no means of assessing whether there is an exact match between the two numbers of hours required to trigger each part of the compensation package.

DECISION ANALYSIS

TIPS & TECHNIQUES

+

78
PRACTICE QUESTIONS

12 Decision Analysis
Format, Purpose & Key Techniques

FORMAT

The decision analysis section of the UKCAT consists of one code comprising symbols/characters, each of which represents a distinct English word.

EXAMPLE CODE		
A = Negative B = Increase C = Use D = Personal	1 = Dwelling 2 = Wood 3 = Tool 4 = Food	∇ = Cold Σ = Large ψ = Full $\div$ = White

Once you have read the code, you must answer 26 questions. These questions fall into three distinct categories:

Category 1: Translation of a given coded message into English
You are given a coded message which contains characters and symbols found in the code table given. You are also given five possible translations, from which you must choose the one which matches the coded message most closely.

Example (Category 1)

Code given: D, BC, ∇4

Option 1: I have increased my consumption of cold food
Option 2: I eat my food cold
Option 3: I like cold food
Option 4: Food is designed to be eaten cold
Option 5: Cold food is nice

In the exam itself, most of the questions would be from this category (approximately 20 out of the 26 questions). The difficulty with this category is in the fact that, though some of the options are obviously wrong, others can be quite close to one another and therefore a degree of interpretation is required.

Category 2: Coding an English sentence

You are given an English sentence and five possible ways of coding it. You must then select amongst the five options the one which constitutes the best way of coding the sentence in question.

Example (Category 2)

Sentence given: My house is less and less white

Option 1: D1❖
Option 2: 1B❖
Option 3: D1, AB, ❖
Option 4: D1, A❖
Option 5: AD1, B❖

In the exam, you can expect 2 to 4 questions of this type, out of a total of 26 questions. The difficulty with this category is that you have to translate several codes to get to the right answer. When the codes are more complex, this can waste valuable time.

Category 3: Identifying missing codes

You are given an English sentence which is difficult to code using the code words provided in the table. You are then given a list of 5 words and must pick one or two (depending on the question) which would be useful additions to the code to help translate the sentence given.

Example (Category 3)

Sentence given: My clothes are too hot in the summer
Choose two words which would be useful additions to the code:

Option 1: Textile
Option 2: Hot
Option 3: Season
Option 4: My
Option 5: Sun

In the exam, you can expect 2 to 4 questions of this type, out of a total of 26 questions. The difficulty lies in the fact that candidates must spend time determining what can be coded using the existing words and what would be really useful to add to the code. This can take some time.

You are given 30 minutes to complete all 26 questions. This includes 1 minute to read some basic instructions. In the "Key Techniques" section which follows, we will provide a range of methods that will enable you to handle all three types of question.

PURPOSE

This exercise tests your ability to make sense of coded information and to exercise your judgement when the information is presented in a non-obvious manner. In some cases, the translation of the code will not match exactly any of the options on offer and you will need to weigh all available options to determine the most suitable.

This replicates situations that you will encounter in the course of your career as a doctor. For example:

- When taking a medical history from a patient, the information may be presented in a format which is not natural to you (but makes sense to the patient).

- When talking to colleagues from other specialties to yours, you may come across information which is communicated in a way that they understand but which, on your side, requires interpretation.

- As a doctor, you will read papers based on research carried out by others, in which the conclusions are unclear or not explicitly stated. You will need to draw your own conclusions in order to determine the extent to which the findings can be applied to your clinical practice.

- In the course of your dealings with other colleagues, people will make assumptions that you are aware of a number of facts and the manner with which they communicate with you will reflect this. You will therefore need to interpret the information required in the best manner that you can.

KEY TECHNIQUES

Category 1 questions: Translating a given code into English

Category 1 questions constitute 80% of all decision analysis questions. It is therefore crucial that you learn to handle these well. In this section we set out a number of techniques which will help you save time and will stop you from falling into common traps. There is more than one way to approach these questions and therefore, whilst we would encourage you to use the techniques set out in this section, you should use the practice questions which follow and the mock exam to develop the approach with which you feel most comfortable.

First step: Translate literally

Translate the code given literally, using the words given in the table. Using the example on the previous page:

D   = Personal
BC   = Increase Use
∇4   = Cold Food

As much as possible, try to keep together the words which are placed together in the coded message; otherwise you will end up with a different translation. For example, in the example above, the "B" is stuck to the "C", and the "∇" is stuck to the "4". This means that these words go together.

Second step: Interpret the result intuitively

Try to make sense of the code in your head to see if you can guess intuitively what this may be about. At this stage, you may want to avoid looking at the possible answers on offer so as not to be unnecessarily influenced. Looking at the above translation, we could interpret this literally as: "I increase my use of cold food".

Third step: Consider the options to see which matches your intuition

The five options offered in this case were:

Option 1: I have increased my consumption of cold food
Option 2: I eat my food cold
Option 3: I like cold food
Option 4: Food is designed to be eaten cold
Option 5: Cold food is nice

- Option 1: I have increased my consumption of cold food
  This seems to be a close match for our intuitive translation "I increase my use of cold food". However, we must make absolutely sure that there is no better option.

- Option 2: I eat my food cold
  This does not make use of the word "Increase". It merely states that the person eats the food cold. Therefore it is not an appropriate translation.

- Option 3: I like cold food
  The original message does not contain the idea of "like". In addition, this translation does not use the word "Increase".

- Option 4: Food is designed to be eaten cold
  This translation does not make use of the word "Personal" or "Increase".

- Option 5: Cold food is nice
  Same issue as for Option 4. In addition, the original message does not mention anything about being "nice".

On balance, Option 1 is therefore the best option.

All code words contained in the coded message must be present in the answer

If you find an option which introduces new concepts (e.g. personalises an answer with "I" when the code is general, or introduces a notion of past or future when the code does not explicitly say so), then it is probably a wrong option.

Watch out for interpretations

For example, the words "Metal Instrument" could equally be translated as "Metal bar", "Key", "Trombone" or any other metallic instrument depending on the context. Although all these words introduce new ideas into the text, they are just extrapolations of an original idea which make a basic code fit into a real-life context. Similarly, the code "Expert Science" could be translated as "Science Teacher" or "Scientist", and the words "Water Container" could be translated as "Water Jug" or "Water Tower", or even

"Sink". All these interpretations are acceptable <u>if, all things considered, there is nothing closer to the original coded message</u>.

Look out for small deviations from the original coded message
In 90% of cases, the incorrect options offered are very close to the correct option and only have a small variation. This includes:

- Words being grouped differently. For example, the code "(Personal Small Man), Acquire, Dwelling" can be translated as "My son is buying a house", whereas "(Personal Man), Acquire, Small, Dwelling" would mean "My husband is buying a small house". This trick is often used in the exam.

- Words being used in the plural in the coded message, but in the singular in the translation, or vice versa. There are cases though where this may be acceptable; for example when the text uses the word "Man" to mean men in general.

- A notion of future or past being introduced or taken out. For example, the coded message may contain the code for "Future" but the translation is in the present tense. There are cases where this may be acceptable depending on the other options (e.g. if "Personal Past Reduce Food Consumption" should be "I have reduced my food consumption" but could be interpreted as "I eat less food" too). Much will depend on the other options available. If one of the options were "In the past, I used to eat less", then this would be more suitable.

- The notion of "Personal" being used in multiple contexts. Often the code word "Personal" is used to mean "I", but can be used in conjunction with other words to take on different meanings. For example, "Plural Personal" can mean "We" or "My friends", whilst "Opposite Personal" can mean "Others".

- The concepts of "Opposite" and "Negative" being used ambiguously. For example, "Opposite Full" can intuitively be interpreted as meaning "empty", but it could also mean "Not full", which is not the same as "empty". The phrase "not full" would be better translated as "Negative Full" but some codes are loosely used or, in fact, the table of codes may not contain the word "Negative". When there is contention as to how such a phrase should be best translated, see if there is another option with a more accurate translation and compare the other points of divergence to determine which, overall, is closest to the original message. Similarly, "Opposite Always" would normally be interpreted as "Never" but, depending on the context and the other options available, could also be interpreted as "Sometimes". Technically though, the word "Sometimes" would be best coded as "Negative Always".

- Using the "least extrapolation" concept. There will be cases where none of the answers are an exact match (otherwise it would be too easy). When this happens, eliminate all the answers which are missing the elements contained in the coded message and, out of the remaining answers, choose those which require the least interpretation. For example, if the code is "Personal, Reduce, Food, Consumption", then the option "I am on a diet" would pose a problem. Indeed, being on a diet does not necessarily mean that you are cutting down on food consumption; it could simply mean that you are eating more or less of one particular type of food. Another option such as "I am cutting down on fatty foods" would also pose a problem since, although it has more words literally matching the original code, it introduces the notion of "fatty foods", which was not there originally. Therefore, on balance, "I am on a diet" is a better match because it retains both the meaning and the generality of the original code.

Category 2 questions: Coding an English sentence
In this exercise, you are given an English sentence and, out of five options, must find the closest matching code. Translating every single option on offer into English could take a while and is therefore not recommended unless the codes contain very few elements.

In almost all cases, the "wrong" options are variations on the theme of the correct option. So, for example, if the correct answer is ""My son has bought a small house", you can bet that the wrong options will translate as something like:
- My sons (i.e. plural) have bought a small house
- My husband has bought a house (i.e. the code for "small" has been moved earlier in the sentence"
- I have bought a small house (i.e. missing the code for "small man")

and so on.

Before you look at the codes on offer, you should therefore get an idea of the codes that you would expect to find in the correct answer and to use the experience gained through your practice to identify where the examiners are likely to make changes in order to confuse you.

If we use the example shown earlier:

Sentence given: My house is less and less white

Option 1: D1❖
Option 2: 1B❖
Option 3: D1, AB, ❖
Option 4: D1, A❖
Option 5: AD1, B❖

Looking at the sentence, we can see that there are two key parts to the sentence:

1 – My house
2 – Less and less white

We would therefore expect some codes such as:
1 – Personal House or Personal Dwelling
2 – Decrease White or Opposite Increase White

This leads us to Option 3.

All other options are variants on this theme. In particular:
Option 1 says "My house is white" (no notion of "less and less").
Option 2 says "Dwelling Increases White" or "The house is/becomes whiter", which does not contain the notion of "I".
Option 4 says "My house is not white", i.e. it omits the "Increase" code.
Option 5 says "Someone else's house becomes whiter", i.e. it places the "Negative" code in the wrong place.

In the exam, all you need to do is find the right answer. You don't have to translate the others. Once you have done a lot of practice in manipulating codes, you will know exactly where the traps are and how examiners tweak the messages to test your logic. It is worth noting that these questions tend to come up towards the end of the decision analysis test, by which time you are familiar enough with the code (having done 20 translations already) to be able to translate sentences the other way round off the top of your head.

Category 3: Identifying missing codes

In this exercise, you must pick out one or two additional code elements from a list of five, which would be useful to translate a given sentence. In the list of five options, three will either be not needed or could be translated using current code words. The easiest way to handle this type of exercise is to split the sentence into its key components and to see how each could be translated. Using the example shown earlier:

Sentence given: My clothes are too hot in the summer
Choose two words which would be useful additions to the code:

Option 1: Textile
Option 2: Hot
Option 3: Season
Option 4: My
Option 5: Sun

One can see that the sentence contains three concepts:
1 – My clothes
2 – Too hot
3 – Summer

"My clothes" will make use of the "Personal" code and therefore we don't need a new code for "My". However, we have nothing to translate the concept of "clothes". Therefore, having the word "Textile" would be useful.

In the code, we have a word for "Cold". Therefore we can translate "hot" as "Negative Cold". This leaves us with the need to translate "Summer", which we could translate as "Hot season"; this means we also need the code for "Season". Note that we could also translate "Summer" as "Sun season" but that would mean having to add "Sun" and this would make it three words instead of two.

Practise, practise, practise

This type of test becomes much easier once you have done dozens of questions and understand where the traps can be. Practising with the questions that follow and those available on the UKCAT website will help you gain confidence and will enable you to recognise quickly the different traps laid out for you by the examiners.

13 Decision Analysis Practice Questions

This section contains 5 codes, for which there are between 11 and 19 different questions, totalling 78 practice questions, i.e. the equivalent of 3 full exams. These questions are designed to help you develop an awareness of the different techniques and tips mentioned in the previous section and span the different types of questions and levels of difficulty that you may encounter in the exam.

If you have already practised for decision analysis exercises through other means, you may wish to practise these questions in real time, in which case you should aim to complete each set of questions as follows:

Code 1: 19 questions in 21 minutes
Code 2: 17 questions in 19 minutes
Code 3: 17 questions in 19 minutes
Code 4: 14 questions in 16 minutes
Code 5: 11 questions in 13 minutes

If, however, you prefer to use these 78 practice questions to develop your awareness of the various difficulties that you may encounter throughout the decision analysis test and to build up your skills and confidence, I would suggest that you take your time to do the first 3 codes, checking the answers as you go along. As you progress towards the latter exercises, you should try to answer questions more quickly, the aim being to be able to answer each individual question in approximately 1 minute once you feel more confident.

The answers to all questions, together with explanations, can be found from page 233 onwards.

Once you have practised answering all 78 questions, you should be ready to confront the mock exam which features at the back of this book and replicates the actual exam's format (i.e. 1 code with 26 questions). You may want to wait until you have practised all sections in this book before going ahead with the mock exam.

DA 1 Practice	PRACTICE CODE 1

CODE 1

A = Opposite	1 = Individual	α = Small
B = Increase	2 = Take	Ω = Cold
C = Positive	3 = Season	λ = Difficult
D = Plural	4 = Thought	Δ = Short
E = Future	5 = Rest	π = Other
F = Seldom	6 = Situation	ω = Legal
G = Combine	7 = Sun	σ = Blue
H = Personal	8 = Air	ψ = Solid
J = Impose	9 = Transportation	Σ = Liquid
	10 = Temper	
	11 = Difficulty	
	12 = Body	
	13 = Relationship	
	14 = Time	
	15 = Repair	
	16 = Quarter	
	17 = Parent	

What is the best interpretation of the following coded messages?

Q1.1:   D(λ,6), F, 1

     A. We rarely face difficult situations
     B. One can feel lonely when dealing with problems
     C. We rarely deal with problems on our own
     D. Troubles come only once
     E. Troubles rarely come on their own

Q1.2:   7, (D11, 12)

☐ **A.** It can be difficult to get a tan
☐ **B.** The sun can cause serious harm to the body
☐ **C.** I don't tan easily
☐ **D.** My skin is sensitive to the sun
☐ **E.** The sun can affect many people

Q1.3:   B(8,9), Ω3

☐ **A.** Air pressure increases when it gets cold
☐ **B.** The air temperature is getting colder
☐ **C.** People breathe more heavily in the winter
☐ **D.** Cold fronts cause stronger winds
☐ **E.** Winds are stronger in the winter

Q1.4:   1AC4, (4, 9, π)

☐ **A.** I feel bad when I think about other people
☐ **B.** Mind-reading can have negative consequences
☐ **C.** I think that telepathy is ludicrous
☐ **D.** I can't stand thinking about other people
☐ **E.** Others often misread my mind

Q1.5:   (A,11), (9, Δ14) $\psi(\sigma, \Sigma)$

☐ **A.** Blue blood is transmitted from generation to generation
☐ **B.** Ice can only be transported for short distances
☐ **C.** Black ice only stays on the road for short periods of time
☐ **D.** Ice melts quickly on the road
☐ **E.** Ice can easily be transported for short periods of time

Q1.6:   D(λ4), B, D(λ6)

☐ **A.** Difficult situations increase pessimism
☐ **B.** Pessimists always overreact in difficult situations
☐ **C.** Pessimists are more likely to run into problems
☐ **D.** Pessimists lead harder lives
☐ **E.** It is difficult to think clearly when you have problems

CODE 1		
A = Opposite	1 = Individual	α = Small
B = Increase	2 = Take	Ω = Cold
C = Positive	3 = Season	λ = Difficult
D = Plural	4 = Thought	Δ = Short
E = Future	5 = Rest	π = Other
F = Seldom	6 = Situation	ω = Legal
G = Combine	7 = Sun	σ = Blue
H = Personal	8 = Air	ψ = Solid
J = Impose	9 = Transportation	Σ = Liquid
	10 = Temper	
	11 = Difficulty	
	12 = Body	
	13 = Relationship	
	14 = Time	
	15 = Repair	
	16 = Quarter	
	17 = Parent	

Q1.7:   **D(Aα,1,9), Bλ(2,8)**

- [ ] **A.** Big cars pollute more
- [ ] **B.** A lorry pollutes more than a car
- [ ] **C.** Cars used to pollute more
- [ ] **D.** Car are responsible for most of the pollution
- [ ] **E.** Coaches pollute more

Q1.8:   **(7,3), BC(D4)**

- [ ] **A.** People feel better in the summer
- [ ] **B.** I feel better when the sun is out
- [ ] **C.** I much prefer going on holiday in the summer
- [ ] **D.** Everyone enjoys thinking about summer
- [ ] **E.** I increasingly feel good in the summer

Q1.9:   1, 11, 5(12,4), (3,5)

☐ **A.** Holidays are not restful
☐ **B.** I can't think clearly at the weekend
☐ **C.** I have trouble relaxing when I am on holiday
☐ **D.** I find Christmas really stressful
☐ **E.** Going on holiday is not always the best way to relax

Q1.10:   Ω3, D(AE,8,9), 11(2,8)

☐ **A.** In winter, old planes have trouble taking off
☐ **B.** In the past, planes could not take off in icy conditions
☐ **C.** Planes do not fly easily in icy conditions
☐ **D.** Old people find it hard to breathe on cold planes
☐ **E.** It is difficult to recycle cold air in old planes

Q1.11:   ω13D1, B(12,14)

☐ **A.** Married people live longer
☐ **B.** Increasingly, old people are getting married
☐ **C.** Married couples are fatter
☐ **D.** Bigamists spend more time with their wives
☐ **E.** People get married later in life

Q1.12:   D3, B(11,12,15)

☐ **A.** It is difficult to receive treatment in the summer
☐ **B.** The older you get, the more difficult it becomes to heal
☐ **C.** Winter increases rheumatisms
☐ **D.** It took me several years to heal
☐ **E.** Old injuries are harder to mend

Q1.13:   AJ, 5, AE, (AΔ9)

☐ **A.** It is recommended to take a nap before a long journey
☐ **B.** No one is forced to remain still during a long trip
☐ **C.** It wasn't compulsory to book a cabin for the long night on the train
☐ **D.** You should have stopped halfway
☐ **E.** In the past, it was impossible to find a hotel so far away

CODE 1		
A = Opposite	1 = Individual	α = Small
B = Increase	2 = Take	Ω = Cold
C = Positive	3 = Season	λ = Difficult
D = Plural	4 = Thought	Δ = Short
E = Future	5 = Rest	π = Other
F = Seldom	6 = Situation	ω = Legal
G = Combine	7 = Sun	σ = Blue
H = Personal	8 = Air	ψ = Solid
J = Impose	9 = Transportation	Σ = Liquid
	10 = Temper	
	11 = Difficulty	
	12 = Body	
	13 = Relationship	
	14 = Time	
	15 = Repair	
	16 = Quarter	
	17 = Parent	

Q1.14:   **DH, π16, AE(7,3)**

☐ **A.** They saw the last quarter of the moon
☐ **B.** We moved out last summer
☐ **C.** Sunny places attract foreign tourists
☐ **D.** We are visiting the historic centre whilst it is sunny
☐ **E.** Summer is a nice time to visit foreign countries

Q1.15:   **GD4(H, HD13), B4**

☐ **A.** Sharing problems with friends often feels good
☐ **B.** My friends are there for me
☐ **C.** I enjoy sharing ideas with my best friend
☐ **D.** It's good to talk
☐ **E.** Brainstorming with my colleagues increases creativity

Q1.16: Which code would best translate the following message: "Relations between school and parents are often tense"?

A. 13, [D17, (α1,16)], AF, λ
B. AF, 11, G (17, α1, A5)
C. 13 (Aα1, α1, 16), λ
D. AF, λ6(D17, α1)
E. (4, 16), AF, λ13, D17

Q1.17: Which would be the most useful two additional codes to convey this message: "You have few minutes to make up your mind in an emergency"?

A. Urgent
B. Mind
C. Minute
D. You
E. Decision

Q1.18: Which would be the most useful two additional codes to convey this message: "The Earth revolves around the Sun in one year"?

A. Sphere
B. Around
C. Year
D. Mars
E. One

Q1.19: Which would be the most useful two additional codes to convey this message: "My blood flows faster when I am angry"?

A. Travel
B. Red
C. Anger
D. Bad
E. Speed

DA 2 Practice	PRACTICE CODE 2

CODE 2

A = Contrary	1 = People	α = Small
B = All	2 = Effect	Ω = Good
C = Plural	3 = Substance	γ = Important
D = Extreme	4 = Health	Σ = Legal
E = Generally	5 = Silence	ε = Severe
F = Only	6 = Use	Δ = Big
G = Add	7 = Animal	η = Able
H = Reflective	8 = Detriment	π = Feminine
J = Other	9 = Alcohol	λ = Strong
K = Less	10 = Illness	
L = Negative	11 = Intensity	
	12 = Tolerant	
	13 = Look	
	14 = Siblings	
	15 = Parent	
	16 = Child	
	17 = Love	
	18 = Listen	

What is the best interpretation of the following coded messages?

Q2.1: 6(AΩ, 3), λ(4,8)

☐ A. Taking too much cocaine can deteriorate health
☐ B. Many fake medical remedies are very bad for health
☐ C. Taking narcotics is very harmful
☐ D. The use of medicine can be very prejudicial to health
☐ E. Taking strong medicines makes me feel ill

Q2.2: AB(AΣ, 3), Σ6, 2(K, 10)

- [ ] **A.** No poison is used legally
- [ ] **B.** Some illegal drugs are used lawfully for the purpose of medical treatment
- [ ] **C.** Some narcotics are believed to be good for use as medication
- [ ] **D.** Some poisons are legal
- [ ] **E.** Not all legal poisons can be used as medication

Q2.3: C (Dα7) AΩ2(1)

- [ ] **A.** Many people are scared of small animals
- [ ] **B.** People catch diseases from insects
- [ ] **C.** Mosquitoes can infect you with malaria
- [ ] **D.** Owning several pets can be detrimental to health
- [ ] **E.** Small insects can be squashed by humans

Q2.4: 11, A5, ε2(1,4)

- [ ] **A.** People can become seriously ill by listening to loud music
- [ ] **B.** Too much exposure to noise can deteriorate people's hearing ability
- [ ] **C.** Quiet music can be beneficial to people's health
- [ ] **D.** Loud noises increase people's deafness
- [ ] **E.** I feel severely unwell when I hear loud music

Q2.5: LB(DΔ,1), (H,13), (F,Δ)

- [ ] **A.** Some obese people don't look as overweight as they are
- [ ] **B.** Not everyone sees obese people as overweight
- [ ] **C.** Only overweight people watch their weight
- [ ] **D.** Some obese people see themselves as being only overweight
- [ ] **E.** Some obese people only fancy other obese people

CODE 2		
A = Contrary	1 = People	α = Small
B = All	2 = Effect	Ω = Good
C = Plural	3 = Substance	γ = Important
D = Extreme	4 = Health	Σ = Legal
E = Generally	5 = Silence	ε = Severe
F = Only	6 = Use	Δ = Big
G = Add	7 = Animal	η = Able
H = Reflective	8 = Detriment	π = Feminine
J = Other	9 = Alcohol	λ = Strong
K = Less	10 = Illness	
L = Negative	11 = Intensity	
	12 = Tolerant	
	13 = Look	
	14 = Siblings	
	15 = Parent	
	16 = Child	
	17 = Love	
	18 = Listen	

Q2.6: (LB1), D(A12), (Aη, 1)

☐ **A.** Many disabled people don't tolerate their handicap
☐ **B.** People are not very tolerant towards the disabled
☐ **C.** Some people find it impossible to accept the disabled
☐ **D.** Intolerant people are unable to deal with others
☐ **E.** Many people are not able to show any intolerance

Q2.7: 1(DH17), (EA17), (CJ)

☐ **A.** Self-important people often don't like others
☐ **B.** People don't tend to like those who are vain
☐ **C.** Famous lovers can be arrogant
☐ **D.** People who enjoy reflecting are not very sociable
☐ **E.** Self-importance will not bring you love

Q2.8: **17, 14, E, AKΔ(17,J1)**

☐ **A.** Having brothers and sisters tends to make you love others more easily
☐ **B.** Brotherly love is not always compatible with friendship
☐ **C.** Big brothers generally develop better friendships
☐ **D.** Brotherly love is often stronger than friendship
☐ **E.** The more obese siblings generally develop better friendships

Q2.9: **C16(L14), FH(13,18)**

☐ **A.** Children don't listen to their siblings
☐ **B.** Children with no siblings are selfish
☐ **C.** Some children have siblings who can't hear or see
☐ **D.** Children with siblings can't hear themselves talk
☐ **E.** Children with no siblings don't pay attention to what others say or do

Q2.10: **(AC), (π15), (λ,ε)2(16)**

☐ **A.** Single mothers are strict disciplinarians
☐ **B.** Children with only one mother are better raised
☐ **C.** Girls are better raised in single-parent families
☐ **D.** No mother raises her child well
☐ **E.** The presence of a grandmother influences the development of a child

Q2.11: **(7, 6), (1, 4), (8, 7)**

☐ **A.** Animal testing for cosmetic reasons cannot be tolerated
☐ **B.** Animals involved in experiments get hurt
☐ **C.** Vets sometimes harm animals
☐ **D.** Animals used in healthcare research suffer
☐ **E.** Humans using animals for healthcare research hurt them

CODE 2		
A = Contrary	1 = People	α = Small
B = All	2 = Effect	Ω = Good
C = Plural	3 = Substance	γ = Important
D = Extreme	4 = Health	Σ = Legal
E = Generally	5 = Silence	ε = Severe
F = Only	6 = Use	Δ = Big
G = Add	7 = Animal	η = Able
H = Reflective	8 = Detriment	π = Feminine
J = Other	9 = Alcohol	λ = Strong
K = Less	10 = Illness	
L = Negative	11 = Intensity	
	12 = Tolerant	
	13 = Look	
	14 = Siblings	
	15 = Parent	
	16 = Child	
	17 = Love	
	18 = Listen	

Q2.12:   **(B, L13, 1) γ(6, 7)**

☐ A. A sizeable number of blind people have dogs
☐ B. Not everyone can look after pets
☐ C. Animals are used to not seeing people
☐ D. Blind animals are of no use to people
☐ E. All blind people should use a guide dog

Q2.13:   **(λ2, 4, 3), [L(Aλ), CJ2]**

☐ A. Strong drugs generally don't have side effects
☐ B. Drugs' side effects should not be ignored
☐ C. Side effects affect patients substantially
☐ D. The side effects of a potent drug are not negligible
☐ E. All strong drugs have side effects

Q2.14: Which code would best translate the following message: "Alcoholism amongst women is a strong taboo"?

A. $(\varepsilon, \pi, 9, 6)$, (D,5)
B. 1, (L, 12), $(\pi, 9, 6)$
C. ε(C, π, 1), E(9, 6)
D. $\lambda 9$, $\varepsilon 2$, $\pi 1$
E. (9,6), 8, $\pi 1$

Q2.15: Which code would best translate the following message: "Laws protecting humans are often against the interests of animals"?

A. $(C\Sigma)$, $(\Omega 2, C7)$, E(L2, 1)
B. $(C\Sigma)$, $2(\Omega 1)$, E(L2, C7)
C. $(C\Sigma)$, $(\Omega 2, A7)$, E(L2, C7)
D. $(C\Sigma)$, $(\Omega 2, 1)$, E(L2, C7)
E. $(C\Sigma)$, $(\Omega 2, 1)$, E($\Omega 2$, C7)

Q2.16: Which code would best translate the following message: "The use of animal tissue for cosmetic purposes is legal"?

A. $6(7,3)$ $(\pi 3)$, Σ
B. $6 (\Omega 13,7)$, Σ
C. $(7,3)$, $(\Sigma,6)(\Omega 13)$
D. $(\Sigma, 7) 6 (\Omega 13,3)$
E. $6(7,3) (\Omega 13,6, \pi 1) \gamma$

Q2.17: Which would be the most useful <u>two additional codes</u> to convey this message: "The prolonged use of alcohol modifies personal physical appearance"?

A. Time
B. Long
C. Different
D. Personal
E. Physical

215

DA 3 Practice	PRACTICE CODE 3

CODE 3

A = Train	α = Fast	1 = Opposite
B = Car	β = Safe	2 = Plural
C = Plane	γ = Cheap	3 = Compare
D = Taxi	Δ = Efficient	4 = Increase
E = Bus	ε = Comfortable	5 = Combine
F = Coach	Σ = Convenient	6 = Circumstance
G = Road	Ω = Sick	7 = Possibility
H = Travel	λ = Always	8 = Personal
K = Business	π = New	9 = Feeling
L = Boat		10 = Acquire
M = Ticket		
N = Outlet		
P = Happiness		

What is the best interpretation of the following coded messages?

Q3.1: (HE, 1ε), 3(HD)

☐ A. A taxi ride is more comfortable than a bus ride
☐ B. Business trips are less comfortable by bus than by taxi
☐ C. A taxi ride does not compare to a bus ride
☐ D. Business trips are more comfortable by bus than by taxi
☐ E. Taxis are often more comfortable than buses

Q3.2: 6(BH) 8, 9, Ω

☐ A. Car travel can make me sick
☐ B. Travelling in a car can make me sick
☐ C. Car travel leads to car sickness
☐ D. Driving makes me feel sick
☐ E. I feel sick when I travel in a car

Q3.3: **(HA, Σ), 3HF, 6K**

☐ **A.** For business trips, taking a train is more convenient than taking a coach
☐ **B.** Coach travel is less convenient than train travel
☐ **C.** Travelling on trains in business class is more convenient than taking a coach
☐ **D.** Business coaches find train travel more convenient
☐ **E.** Conducting business on a train is easier than on a coach

Q3.4: **5(2E), (7,4α), 3(1, 2, C)**

☐ **A.** Several buses travel faster than planes
☐ **B.** Taking a series of several buses can be faster than taking one plane
☐ **C.** Taking a plane can be faster than taking a bus
☐ **D.** Travelling to the airport by bus is possibly the fastest way
☐ **E.** It is possible to travel fast by combining bus and plane travel

Q3.5: **H5(D,E), 1α, 3(HB)**

☐ **A.** Travelling by bus or taxi takes longer than by car
☐ **B.** A journey consisting of a taxi ride followed by a bus ride normally takes longer than a car journey
☐ **C.** It is faster to travel by car than by combining taxi and bus rides
☐ **D.** It is quicker not to travel by taxi or bus
☐ **E.** Travelling by taxi and bus in the same journey is faster than travelling by car

Q3.6: **6(1, K), 1, 8, B**

☐ **A.** When business was not going well, I often borrowed a friend's car
☐ **B.** I use my own car for business purposes
☐ **C.** I don't have a company car
☐ **D.** I never drive alone on business trips
☐ **E.** When I go on holiday, I rent a car

CODE 3		
A = Train	α = Fast	1 = Opposite
B = Car	β = Safe	2 = Plural
C = Plane	γ = Cheap	3 = Compare
D = Taxi	Δ = Efficient	4 = Increase
E = Bus	ε = Comfortable	5 = Combine
F = Coach	Σ = Convenient	6 = Circumstance
G = Road	Ω = Sick	7 = Possibility
H = Travel	λ = Always	8 = Personal
K = Business	π = New	9 = Feeling
L = Boat		10 = Acquire
M = Ticket		
N = Outlet		
P = Happiness		

Q3.7: 2E, λH5(2E)

A. Group travel is best done by bus
B. I tend to combine several bus journeys when I travel
C. Several buses often come at once
D. There are always several buses travelling together
E. Travelling together by bus can be fun

Q3.8: γ(HL, 1K), 5(α, Σ), 1λε

A. Cruises are sometimes cheap, fast and convenient but not always comfortable
B. Pleasure boat trips are sometimes cheap, fast and convenient but are rarely comfortable
C. Cheap yachts can be fast and convenient but are never comfortable
D. Cheap cruises are fast and convenient but not always comfortable
E. I don't often travel on cheap boats for business purposes as they are often uncomfortable

Q3.9: **(5, 2, M), 1λ, 4γ, (3, 2, M)**

☐ **A.** Buying a season ticket is not always cheaper than buying several tickets

☐ **B.** Buying one return ticket is sometimes cheaper than buying two single tickets

☐ **C.** The price of season tickets does not always increase by more than the price of individual tickets

☐ **D.** Discounts are often available for those who travel in groups

☐ **E.** Large families travel more cheaply than individuals

Q3.10: **HM5(C,B), (7, 4, γ, Δ), 6(KHN)**

☐ **A.** Combined flight-car tickets are often cheaper

☐ **B.** It can be cheaper and more efficient to purchase a fly-drive ticket from a travel agency

☐ **C.** Organised tours are possibly cheaper than individual trips

☐ **D.** Travel agencies can offer better deals on fly-drive holidays

☐ **E.** I prefer to buy my cheap fly-drive tickets from the more organised travel agencies

Q3.11: **(8, π, 9), (8AMN), 1β**

☐ **A.** I think that the train station they built recently is unsafe

☐ **B.** I was recently assaulted at my local train station

☐ **C.** I am starting to feel that my local train station is unsafe

☐ **D.** Local trains have recently been reported as unsafe

☐ **E.** I have always felt unsafe at my local train station

Q3.12: **Which code would best translate the following message: "One journey sometimes requires several tickets"?**

☐ **A.** 1, 2 , 6H, λ2M

☐ **B.** 8, H, 2, M

☐ **C.** 2, 6H, (1, 7), 2M

☐ **D.** 1, 2 , 6H, 7, 5(2M)

☐ **E.** 7(1, 2, M), 6(2H)

CODE 3		
A = Train	α = Fast	1 = Opposite
B = Car	β = Safe	2 = Plural
C = Plane	γ = Cheap	3 = Compare
D = Taxi	Δ = Efficient	4 = Increase
E = Bus	ε = Comfortable	5 = Combine
F = Coach	Σ = Convenient	6 = Circumstance
G = Road	Ω = Sick	7 = Possibility
H = Travel	λ = Always	8 = Personal
K = Business	π = New	9 = Feeling
L = Boat		10 = Acquire
M = Ticket		
N = Outlet		
P = Happiness		

Q3.13: Which code would best translate the following message: "I feel sicker when I travel by bus than by boat"?

A. 6(EH), 8, 4(9Ω), 3, 6(LH)
B. 6(EH), 4, Ω, 3, 6L
C. (8, λ, 9, Ω), H, 3 (E,L)
D. 6(FH), 8, 4, ε, 3, 6 (LH)
E. 8(9, Ω) 6(EH) 3L

Q3.14: Which code would best translate the following message: "My friends like sailing"?

A. (2, 8), (1, 9, P), 6 (HL)
B. (2, 8), (9, P), 2L
C. (2, 8), (λ, β, 9), 6(LH)
D. (2, 8), λHL
E. (2, 8), (9, P), 6(HL)

Q3.15: Which would be the most useful <u>two additional codes</u> to convey this message: "It is possible to get cheap tickets at the last minute"?

☐ **A.** Buy
☐ **B.** Late
☐ **C.** Can
☐ **D.** Purchase
☐ **E.** Time

Q3.16: Which would be the most useful <u>two additional codes</u> to convey this message: "Boat cruises abroad can be dangerous for your health"?

☐ **A.** Territory
☐ **B.** Dangerous
☐ **C.** Other
☐ **D.** Trip
☐ **E.** Health

Q3.17: Which would be the most useful <u>two additional codes</u> to convey this message: "The construction of a new runway makes me feel angry"?

☐ **A.** Build
☐ **B.** Anger
☐ **C.** Makes
☐ **D.** Airport
☐ **E.** Runway

DA 4 Practice	PRACTICE CODE 4

CODE 4		
A = Amplify	1 = Population	α = Legal
B = Same	2 = Idea	β = Level
C = Always	3 = Large	γ = Free
D = Future	4 = Intense	δ = Positive
E = Opposite	5 = Pool	π = Full
F = Consequence	6 = Food	σ = Calm
G = Negative	7 = Fluid	
	8 = Money	
	9 = Work	
	10 = Hate	
	11 = Person	
	12 = Path	
	13 = Event	
	14 = Discord	
	15 = Traffic	
	16 = Departure	
	17 = Rise	
	18 = Farm	

What is the best interpretation of the following coded messages?

Q4.1:   3, 16, E9, FE(15,7)

    A. Mass redundancies provoke strikes that cripple the country

    B. Commuters cause traffic congestion

    C. Heavy holiday departures cause traffic jams

    D. Getting stuck in traffic whilst going on holiday can be stressful

    E. Long holidays always involve traffic jams

Q4.2: **10, E(B11), GC, FA14**

- [ ] **A.** Hatred of others sometimes leads to war
- [ ] **B.** Selfishness sometimes paves the way for conflict
- [ ] **C.** People who hate others never agree with anyone
- [ ] **D.** It's often the same people who are looking for trouble
- [ ] **E.** Most people hate those who look for trouble

Q4.3: **(E17), 18, F(Eπ, 6), (3, 1)**

- [ ] **A.** Smaller farms produce better food for customers
- [ ] **B.** Agricultural decline causes lack of food in cities
- [ ] **C.** Poor harvesting provoked starvation for the whole population
- [ ] **D.** It takes fewer farmers to produce enough food for cities
- [ ] **E.** The decreasing number of farms is not sufficient to fulfil the increasing need in food in growing cities

Q4.4: **(5, 2), FA9**

- [ ] **A.** Brainstorming encourages productivity
- [ ] **B.** I work better at the poolside
- [ ] **C.** I think better after a good swim.
- [ ] **D.** I have the idea of building a fishpond
- [ ] **E.** Leisure times help people work harder

Q4.5: **(E3, 15) F, 17, (Eα, 15)**

- [ ] **A.** There aren't many illegal goods around
- [ ] **B.** Traffickers control the food market
- [ ] **C.** It is illegal to close down small markets
- [ ] **D.** It is illegal to drive on market days
- [ ] **E.** Low supply leads to the development of a black market

CODE 4		
A = Amplify	1 = Population	α = Legal
B = Same	2 = Idea	β = Level
C = Always	3 = Large	γ = Free
D = Future	4 = Intense	δ = Positive
E = Opposite	5 = Pool	π = Full
F = Consequence	6 = Food	σ = Calm
G = Negative	7 = Fluid	
	8 = Money	
	9 = Work	
	10 = Hate	
	11 = Person	
	12 = Path	
	13 = Event	
	14 = Discord	
	15 = Traffic	
	16 = Departure	
	17 = Rise	
	18 = Farm	

Q4.6:   **(E, π), (9, 6), CF(1, 4, 16)**

- [ ] **A.** Birds migrate to look for food.
- [ ] **B.** Lack of resources always provokes migrations
- [ ] **C.** Displacement of people is often caused by the lack of resources
- [ ] **D.** Farm workers always travel a lot to look for work
- [ ] **E.** Most people go shopping at the weekend

Q4.7:   Eγ(1,9), DE(Eα)

☐ **A.** Slavery will not be abolished
☐ **B.** Some prisons will close in the near future
☐ **C.** Salaried workers are legal
☐ **D.** Slavery will be illegal
☐ **E.** Making prisoners work will no longer be legal

Q4.8:   (1, γ, 9, 18), (A15, E16)

☐ **A.** There are many volunteers on farms
☐ **B.** Pensioners like visiting farms
☐ **C.** More and more people leave farming jobs to work elsewhere as volunteers
☐ **D.** More people are coming to do voluntary work on farms
☐ **E.** Freelance workers will increasingly be accepted in farming jobs

Q4.9:   (15, 12), (3, 14), DCF(Eγ)

☐ **A.** Those who campaign against road building programmes are likely to be jailed
☐ **B.** Arguments against road charges are inconsequential
☐ **C.** Road rage will be rewarded by a prison sentence
☐ **D.** Severely damaging a road will give rise to a fine.
☐ **E.** An argument about travel directions could cost you dear

Q4.10:   7, β(17, E17), FEA, 16, 15

☐ **A.** Tides are slowing down departures
☐ **B.** Boats come and go depending on the tide
☐ **C.** Boats make waves
☐ **D.** Owners need to evacuate the water from their boat before departing
☐ **E.** Boats leave port at high tide and not at low tide

CODE 4		
A = Amplify	1 = Population	α = Legal
B = Same	2 = Idea	β = Level
C = Always	3 = Large	γ = Free
D = Future	4 = Intense	δ = Positive
E = Opposite	5 = Pool	π = Full
F = Consequence	6 = Food	σ = Calm
G = Negative	7 = Fluid	
	8 = Money	
	9 = Work	
	10 = Hate	
	11 = Person	
	12 = Path	
	13 = Event	
	14 = Discord	
	15 = Traffic	
	16 = Departure	
	17 = Rise	
	18 = Farm	

Q4.11:   π, 8, EF, π(3, 2)

- **A.** A lot of money can give you an interesting life
- **B.** Wealthy people are not the more tolerant
- **C.** Wealth has no bearing on intelligence
- **D.** Creativity brings expenses
- **E.** Prosperity sometimes goes with a boring life

Q4.12: **Which code would best translate the following message: "Money does not always make you happy"?**

☐ **A.** 8, F(E, δ, 11)
☐ **B.** 8, EC, F(δ, 11)
☐ **C.** 8, EA, δ, 2
☐ **D.** 17, 8, A4, δ
☐ **E.** (G, 5, 8), EA, δ, 11

Q4.13: **Which would be <u>the most useful additional code</u> to convey this message: "Optimists have a better chance of getting a pay increase"?**

☐ **A.** Optimist
☐ **B.** Pay
☐ **C.** Probability
☐ **D.** Increase
☐ **E.** Happy

Q4.14: **Which would be <u>the two most useful additional codes</u> to convey this message: "Few tribes live high in the rocky mountains"?**

☐ **A.** Few
☐ **B.** High
☐ **C.** Stone
☐ **D.** Tribe
☐ **E.** Live

DA 5 Practice	**PRACTICE CODE 5**

CODE 5

A = Opposite	1 = Master	Σ = Good
B = Increase	2 = Art	Ω = Over
C = Singular	3 = Sound	Δ = Near
D = Past	4 = Person	π = Safe
E = Possibility	5 = Look	
F = Consequence	6 = Save	
	7 = Start	
	8 = Stone	
	9 = Wood	
	10 = Shift	
	11 = Building	
	12 = Instrument	
	13 = Show	
	14 = Period	
	15 = Weight	
	16 = Stick	
	17 = Light	
	18 = Water	

Q5.1: **1(10, 16), F(AC, 12, 7)**

- A. The karate master starts teaching traditional weapons
- B. The experienced boatman starts rowing with two paddles
- C. The commander is at the helm and is shouting orders to start lowering the sails
- D. As the conductor moves his baton, the orchestra starts playing
- E. The shepherd can play several instruments

Q5.2:   2, 11, (AC)(Σ13), D14

- [ ] **A.** It is interesting to show how this piece of art was made.
- [ ] **B.** This art gallery never displayed any nice paintings
- [ ] **C.** Architecture from antiquity can be seen in many sites
- [ ] **D.** Every year, I visited a museum and saw nice exhibitions
- [ ] **E.** The museum used to present good exhibitions

Q5.3:   Ω,15, F(AE, 10, 8, 2)

- [ ] **A.** The marble sculpture can't be removed; it's too heavy!
- [ ] **B.** I ate too much; I can't visit another monument
- [ ] **C.** This heavy obelisk is impossible to displace
- [ ] **D.** Removing a big piece of jewellery is quite impossible
- [ ] **E.** I can't take it upon myself to get rid of this sculpture

Q5.4:   4, 9, 12, ΔAD, C1

- [ ] **A.** The woodcutter is my neighbour's only teacher
- [ ] **B.** The violin player will soon be a soloist
- [ ] **C.** This string instrument maker will one day make a masterpiece
- [ ] **D.** In the future, craftsmen will work with natural materials
- [ ] **E.** This harpist is a promising student,

Q5.5:   8, 14, AC12, (9, 16)

- [ ] **A.** During the Stone Age, many weapons' handles were made of wood
- [ ] **B.** Diamond trade was organised by canoe
- [ ] **C.** During the gold rush, people would make their own tools with wood
- [ ] **D.** When you are stoned, you can feel a bit wooden
- [ ] **E.** Several instruments, such as recorders, are made of wood

CODE 5		
A = Opposite	1 = Master	Σ = Good
B = Increase	2 = Art	Ω = Over
C = Singular	3 = Sound	Δ = Near
D = Past	4 = Person	π = Safe
E = Possibility	5 = Look	
F = Consequence	6 = Save	
	7 = Start	
	8 = Stone	
	9 = Wood	
	10 = Shift	
	11 = Building	
	12 = Instrument	
	13 = Show	
	14 = Period	
	15 = Weight	
	16 = Stick	
	17 = Light	
	18 = Water	

Q5.6:   Ω11, EF, AB9

- A. Excessive urbanisation can lead to deforestation
- B. Building too many houses means too much wood is used
- C. Wood is used less and less to build skyscrapers
- D. Scaffoldings can be made of wood
- E. From the roof, we can hardly see a tree

Q5.7:   (1, 6, D), 5, AC [(D,4, 8), (D, 4, 11)]

A. My teacher checked if we brought dangerous objects in
B. Ancient medicine men used stones and buildings inherited from their ancestors
C. An archaeologist looks at old cemeteries and old cities
D. The first bankers believed in investing in ancient stones and ancient buildings.
E. My first clock was taken from an old building and looked like it was made of stone

Q5.8:   17, 12, BΣ5, 13, 1

A. The gadget demonstrator convinces others that his product is the best
B. A projector makes an artist look better
C. The lighthouse helps boatmen see better
D. Fireworks are more and more beautiful
E. The clown uses a mirror that makes people look good

Q5.9:   1(18, 11), 5, 18, E(Aπ8)

A. The water tower's manager dropped stones into the water
B. I see water falling dangerously from the dam onto rocks
C. An experienced diver scans the sea for dangerous rocks
D. The dangerous mountain is visible from the huge bridge across the bay
E. The captain scans the sea for a possible dangerous rock

Q5.10:   (18, 15)Ω, E, A (π,4)

A. Too much water pressure may endanger people
B. Drinking too much water may be a cause of obesity
C. Giving too much water to a dehydrated person can be dangerous
D. It is impossible to transport water to a drought-suffering nation
E. One should be careful when carrying water

CODE 5		
A = Opposite	1 = Master	Σ = Good
B = Increase	2 = Art	Ω = Over
C = Singular	3 = Sound	Δ = Near
D = Past	4 = Person	π = Safe
E = Possibility	5 = Look	
F = Consequence	6 = Save	
	7 = Start	
	8 = Stone	
	9 = Wood	
	10 = Shift	
	11 = Building	
	12 = Instrument	
	13 = Show	
	14 = Period	
	15 = Weight	
	16 = Stick	
	17 = Light	
	18 = Water	

Q5.11: Which would be <u>the two most useful additional codes</u> to convey this message: "It is never safe to be in an open-air swimming pool during a storm"?

A. Risk
B. Always
C. Lightning
D. Swimming
E. Outside

14 Decision Analysis Answers to Practice Questions

DA1 – PRACTICE CODE 1

Q1.1 – E: Troubles rarely come on their own

D(λ6) = Plural (Difficult Situation)
F = Seldom
1 = Individual

Looking at the other answers:

Answer A: We rarely face difficult situations

The notion of "we" does not feature in the coded message. Also, the combination of "Seldom" and "Individual" in the code suggests that the difficult situations mentioned are not isolated incidents. Answer A introduces the concept of "rarely" which means the opposite.

Answer B: One can feel lonely when dealing with problems

The coded message does not contain the notion of "feeling". It does, however contain the concept of "Seldom" which is not being addressed in this translation. Instead, Answer B simply mentions that "one can feel". This is not strong enough as a translation of "Seldom".

Answer C: We rarely deal with problems on our own

The notions of "we" and of "dealing" do not feature in the coded message.

Answer D: Troubles come only once

This translation is too strong because it introduces the concept of "only" whilst the coded message only mentions "Seldom". Answer E is more accurate in this regard.

Comments

This code can effectively be translated as "Difficult situations are rarely individual". When there are no verbs in the coded message, you can often add "are" or "is" to obtain a basic translation. In this case, you would get: "Difficult situations are rarely individual", which is closely matched by Answer E: "Troubles rarely come on their own". Watch out for answers which add new notions such as "feel" or "deal" in this question. Answer E does introduce the notion of "come" but in this context the word "come" really means "happen" or "are". Bear in mind too that what you must find is not an exact translation, but the closest.

Q1.2 – B: The sun can cause serious harm to the body

7   = Sun
D11, 12   = Plural Difficulty, Body

In this question, the word "Plural" applies to the word "Difficulty" and there is no notion of "Personal" (Code H) or "Individual" (Code 1). Therefore any translation would need to be general.

Looking at the other answers:

Answer A: It can be difficult to get a tan
This answer does not contain any notion of several difficulties.

Answer C: I don't tan easily
The coded message has no notion of "Personal".

Answer D: My skin is sensitive to the sun
The coded message has no notion of "Personal". In addition, there is no mention of the skin in the coded message. This translation does not allow for several difficulties and the fact that the sun is associated with difficulties does not imply that the skin is sensitive anyway.

Answer E: The sun can affect many people
There is no notion of "many people" in the coded message. The plural applies to difficulties.

Comments
Answer B is the best solution because it contains all the concepts present in the coded message, with some extrapolation required in order to associate the concept of "serious harm" to "Plural Difficulty". This may not be entirely accurate but Answer B remains the closest solution out of all five proposed.

Remember that you are not necessarily looking for an exact translation but for the best interpretation.

Q1.3 – E: Winds are stronger in the winter

B(8,9)   = Increase (Air, Transportation)
Ω3   = Cold, Season

This code simply points to a relationship between an increase in air transportation (which could be interpreted as wind) and a cold season (e.g. winter) so Answer E seems the most natural. Looking at the other options:

Answer A: Air pressure increases when it gets cold
There is no notion of "pressure" in the coded message, only of "Transportation", i.e. movement.

Answer B: The air temperature is getting colder
This statement does not make use of the concept of "Transportation", i.e. movement. Also, the notion of "Cold" applies to a season, not to the air.

Answer C: People breathe more heavily in the winter
This statement suits the coded message in many ways as it uses the concepts of increasing air movements and of cold season, but it also has an added notion of "people" which is not included in the coded message. Answer E is therefore closer.

Answer D: Cold fronts cause stronger winds
There is no notion of "causation" in the coded message.

Q1.4 – C: I think that telepathy is ludicrous

1AC4   = Individual Opposite Positive Thought
4, 9, π   = Thought, Transportation, Other

The code has two separate components:
- 1AC4 which can be interpreted as "I think negatively or badly"
- 4, 9, π which can be interpreted as telepathy, mind-reading or any concept of conveying thoughts to others.

As such, Option C is the closest match. Looking at the other options:

Answer A: I feel bad when I think about other people
This answer does not use the concept of transport of thoughts. The thoughts stay within you.

Answer B: Mind-reading can have negative consequences
This does not use the "Personal" concept. Also, the coded message does not mention anything about negative consequences, merely negative thoughts.

Answer D: I can't stand thinking about other people
This does not use the concept of "Transportation", i.e. you keep your thoughts to yourself. The answer "I can't stand telling people what I think" would be a possible answer though, but unfortunately does not feature in the list.

Answer E: Others often misread my mind
The coded message does not contain the notion of "often". This answer also introduces the notion of "misread" which does not feature in the code, the only negative referring to personal thoughts.

Q1.5 – E: Ice can easily be transported for short periods of time

A, 11   = Opposite Difficulty
9, Δ14   = Transportation, Short Time
$\psi(\sigma, \Sigma)$ = Solid (Blue Liquid)

This can literally be translated as "It is not difficult to transport solid blue liquid for a short time", hence Answer E is closest.

Answer A: Blue blood is transmitted from generation to generation
This does not use the concept of "Solid", or "Short Time".

Answer B: Ice can only be transported for short distances
The concept of "only" is not in the coded message. We are told that it is not difficult to transport for a short time, but nothing about long periods of time. Also the concept of "Short Time" is not necessarily equivalent to "short distances" since it can take a long time to travel a short distance.

Answer C: Black ice only stays on the road for short periods of time
This does not use the notion of "Transportation".

Answer D: Ice melts quickly on the road
This does not use the notion of "Transportation" or "Difficulty".

Q1.6 – D: Pessimists lead harder lives

D(λ4)   = Plural (Difficult Thought)
B   = Increase
D(λ6)   = Plural (Difficult Situation)

Why the other answers are not appropriate:

Answer A: Difficult situations increase pessimism
The coded messages suggest that the difficult thoughts (i.e. pessimism) increase the problems, and not the other way round.

Answer B: Pessimists always overreact in difficult situations
The coded message does not contain the concept of "always". As far as "overreact" is concerned, the notion of "Increase" applies to the "Difficult Situations" and not to the "Difficult Thoughts".

Answer C: Pessimists are more likely to run into problems
The words "more likely" imply that this is not always the case. There is no such concept in the coded message.

Answer E: It is difficult to think clearly when you have problems
This answer does not contain the notion of "Increase". It also implies that the problems lead to the difficult thoughts, whereas the coded message actually states the opposite.

Comments
Once you have translated the code literally, try to add a few neutral link words (i.e. words which bind the existing words together but do not alter the meaning). Here we have: "Difficult thoughts increase difficult situations". We could improve this by saying "Having difficult thoughts increases the number (or the size) of problems". Having difficult thoughts can be related to pessimism and, if no other answer provides a closer match, then Answer D is the best option.

Here, the coded message does not contain the notion of "people" and therefore we have had to extrapolate that "Difficult Thoughts" equals "pessimists". Answer D is therefore not a close translation of the coded message, but it is the answer which extrapolates the least, i.e. it offers the closest fit. The others either translate the message the wrong way round or add concepts which totally change the meaning of the message.

Q1.7 – A: Big cars pollute more

D(Aα,1,9) = Plural (Opposite Small, Individual, Transportation)
Bλ(2,8)   = Increase Difficult (Take, Air)

A first adaptation of the above literal translation would be "Big cars make breathing more difficult". But none of the options appear to match this interpretation very closely.

Looking at the other answers:

Answer B: A lorry pollutes more than a car
The coded message does not compare two modes of transport.

Answer C: Cars used to pollute more
The coded message does not talk about cars in the past. This answer also does not use the notion of "Opposite Small", i.e. large.

Answer D: Cars are responsible for most of the pollution
This does not use the notion of "large cars". In addition, the coded message only mentions that breathing is becoming more difficult because of large cars, and not that cars are responsible for most of the pollution.

Answer E: Coaches pollute more
The coded message mentions individual transport. Coaches aren't individual.

Comments
In this exercise, the idea of breathing difficulty has been translated in all possible answers by using the concept of "pollution". Therefore the difference between each of the answers lies mainly in the misinterpretation of the first part of the code.

Q1.8 – A: People feel better in the summer

(7,3)   = Sun, Season
BC(D4)   = Increase Positive (Plural Thought)

Translated literally, this would give "The sun season (i.e. possibly the summer) increases positive thoughts", which Answer A matches closely.

Looking at the other answers:

Answer B: I feel better when the sun is out
This introduces the notion of "I", i.e. something personal, which does not feature in the coded message.

Answer C: I much prefer going on holiday in the summer
The coded message refers to positive thoughts and not holiday. Also, there is no notion of "I" in the message.

Answer D: Everyone enjoys thinking about the summer
This answer does not use the concept of "Increase".

Answer E: I increasingly feel good in the summer
This answer introduces the concept of "I" which does not feature in the message. Answer A is a closer match.

Q1.9 – C: I have trouble relaxing when I am on holiday

1	= Individual
11	= Difficulty
5(12,4)	= Rest (Body, Thought)
(3,5)	= (Season, Rest)

The literal interpretation of the above information would be "I have difficulty relaxing during the season of rest (i.e. holidays/weekend)", which matches Answer C.

Looking at the other answers:

Answer A: Holidays are not restful
This does not contain the notion of "Personal", or the notion of Difficulty. The statement is presented as a certainty.

Answer B: I can't think clearly at the weekend
This uses the concept of "Thought" but not of "Body" or of "Rest".

Answer D: I find Christmas really stressful

This uses all the concepts within the code but the use of the word "really" is superfluous. Also, it narrows the rest season to Christmas, whereas Answer C keeps it at the broad level indicated by the coded message. This answer would be a strong contender if Answer A was not available.

Answer E: Going on holiday is not always the best way to relax

This does not use the notion of "Personal".

Q1.10 – A: In winter, old planes have trouble taking off

Ω3   = Cold Season
D(AE,8,9) = Plural (Opposite Future, Air, Transportation)
11(2,8)   = Difficulty (Take, Air)

This can be interpreted simply as "When it is cold, old planes find it difficult to fly", which would seem to match Answer A fairly closely. We now need to look at the other options to discount them.

Answer B: In the past, planes could not take off in icy conditions

This answer also matches closely the coded message but the notion of "past" is not directly linked to the planes. The message has "Opposite Future", "Air" and "Transportation" all in the same bracket. For Answer B to be more suitable than Answer A, the code would need to have AE "Opposite Future" outside the bracket.

Answer C: Planes do not fly easily in icy conditions

This does not use the concept of "old".

Answer D: Old people find it hard to breathe on cold planes

In the message, "Old" refers to planes and not people. Also, in the message, "Cold" refers to the season and not to the plane.

Answer E: it is difficult to recycle cold air in old planes

The notion of "Cold" applies to the season and not to the air.

Q1.11 – A: Married people live longer

ω13D1   = Legal Relationship Plural Individual
B(12,14) = Increase (Body, Time)

This coded message conveys two central ideas:
- The idea of a legal relationship between at least two people, which could be a business partnership or a marriage, for example.
- The idea of increased body and time, which could be interpreted as spending more time together, or living longer.

In that respect, Answer A fits the code well. However, we need to analyse the other answers to see whether another phrase could be a better fit:

Answer B: Increasingly, old people are getting married
The concept of "Increase (Body, Time)"could, at a stretch, refer to old people. If that were the case then the word "Increasingly" would not be appropriate as the "Increase" concept would already have been used to mean "old".

Answer C: Married couples are fatter
"Increase Body" could indeed mean "fat". However, this does not convey the notion of "Time".

Answer D: Bigamists spend more time with their wives
This answer is also a good match for the coded message. However, it does introduce the concept of "wife" which is not in the original message. All it says is that they spend more time; there is no detail on who with. Note also that the term "Increase" also applies to the word "Body" and not just the word "Time".

Answer E: People get married later in life
The concept of "Increase Time" is present, but not that of "Body".

Comments
This question illustrates, perhaps more than the others, how much the answer relies on interpretation. Many of the above answers would fit if it were not for a bracket in the wrong place. Once you have eliminated the obvious wrong answers, then go back to your basic code and identify the answer which requires the least interpretation or the least amount of new words to be added to make sense of the code.

Q1.12 – B: The older you get, the more difficult it becomes to heal

D3   = Plural Season
B(11,12,15)   = Increase (Difficulty, Body, Repair)

Intuitively, this could be translated as "Several seasons increase the difficulty for the body to get repaired", which fits well the concept conveyed by Answer B. Checking other answers:

Answer A: It is difficult to receive treatment in the summer
The season is not mentioned in the code and therefore the use of "summer" is an extrapolation. Answer B handles the concept of season more generically than Answer A. In addition, this answer does not make use of the notion of "Increase"; it merely points to a difficulty and would have been appropriate if it had mentioned that "it has become harder to receive treatment in the summer".

Answer C: Winter increases rheumatisms
The use of a specific season is an extrapolation of the word "Season". In addition, this answer ignores the concept of "Repair", focusing instead on the increase in the condition rather than the treatment or cure.

Answer D: It took me several years to heal
This answer has a personal touch "It took me" which is not contained in the coded message. In addition, it does not make use of the notion of "Increase".

Answer E: Old injuries are harder to mend
"Increase (Difficulty, Body, Repair)" could correspond to "are harder to mend" and in fact is used in this context within Answer B. The concept of "Plural Season" could be translated as "old" but it would not apply to injuries.

Q1.13 – A: It is recommended to take a nap before a long journey

AJ	= Opposite Impose
5	= Rest
AE	= Opposite Future
A$\triangle$9	= Opposite Short Transportation

This could be translated in several ways, including:
- It is recommended to rest before a long journey (with the "recommendation" corresponding to the "non-imposition".
- It is not compulsory to rest before a long journey.
- In the past, it was recommended to rest during a long journey.

There are several combinations of words which are all used in one way or another in all the options on offer. Therefore, although the Answer A seems to fit the coded message closely, we need to test the other options:

Answer B: No one is forced to remain still during a long trip
This ignores the notion of "Opposite Future".

Answer C: It wasn't compulsory to book a cabin for the long night on the train. This introduces the notions of "night" and "train", which, although valid, are not as close a fit as the notion of "long journey" presented in some of the other options, including Answer A. Also, this answer equates the booking of a cabin with the notion of "Rest". This is valid too but requires more interpretation than other answers require.

Answer D: You should have stopped halfway
This introduces the notion of "you" whereas the coded message is more of a generic nature. Also, there is no notion of "long Transportation".

Answer E: In the past, it was impossible to find a hotel so far away
This does not allow for the concept of "Opposite Impose".

Q1.14 – B: We moved out last summer

DH = Plural Personal

$\pi16$ = Other Quarter

AE(7,3) = Opposite Future (Sun, Season)

The difficulty with this code resides in the fact that it is actually missing a verb and therefore there is room for speculation (and therefore error!). However, many answers can be eliminated in one sweep as follows: the phrase "Plural Personal" is used to denote several people associated with you and therefore could translate into "We" or "My friends". This essentially takes out of circulation Answers A, C and E, none of which make use of the "Plural Personal" concept. This leaves Answer B and Answer D as possibilities, both of which start with "We".

Answer D can also be eliminated because it mentions "whilst it is sunny" when the coded message talks about "Opposite Future (Sun, Season)", i.e. last summer.

To summarise and complement:

Answer A: They saw the last quarter of the moon
"They" does not match with the "Plural Personal" concept. Also, the word "Opposite" is applying to "Future" rather than to "Sun, Season". Even if it applied to "Sun, Season", we would then be left with a Future Moon, which does not necessarily indicate the last quarter.

Answer C: Sunny places attract foreign tourists
No reference to a sun season, only to sunny places. Also, the word "tourists" does not match the "Plural Personal" concept.

Answer D: We are visiting the historic centre whilst it is sunny
The word "historic" comes either from the loose interpretation of "other quarter" (possible, but a bit far-fetched) or from the association of "Opposite Future" to the word "Quarter", which would be incorrect. Answer B is a better fit.

Answer E: Summer is a nice time to visit foreign countries
There is no use of the concept of "Opposite Future", i.e. past. Also there is no relationship to the concept of "Plural Personal".

Q1.15 – E: Brainstorming with my colleagues increases creativity

GD4   = Combine Plural Thought
H, HD13 = Personal, Personal Plural Relationship
B4   = Increase Thoughts

Literally, this would translate as "Sharing different ideas with people close to me increases thoughts". In this regard, Answer E is closest.

Answer A: Sharing problems with friends often feels good
This contains the notion of "combining thoughts" (though introduces the notion of "negativity" with the word "problems"). The words "often" and "good" are not in the coded message. We are simply told that it increases thoughts as opposed to "good thoughts".

Answer B: My friends are there for me
This has no notion of combining personal thoughts with those of others, or of increasing thoughts.

Answer C: I enjoy sharing ideas with my best friend
This introduces the notion of "enjoyment". The concept of "best friend" could be accepted as a translation of "Personal Relationship" but it is plural in the coded message.

Answer D: It's good to talk
This has no notion of increasing thoughts. The concept of "talking" is also ambiguous because it does not necessarily involve sharing thoughts with others. This answer does not use the concept of "Personal and Personal Relationships".

Q1.16 – A: 13, [D17, (α1,16)], AF, λ

Answer A = Relationship [Plural Parent, Small Individual, Quarter] Opposite Seldom, Difficult. This code leaves little ambiguity and is the correct code. The other codes translate as follows:

Answer B: Opposite Seldom, Difficulty, Combine (Parent, Small Individual, Opposite Rest). There is no notion of school in the code and it suggests instead that the disagreements are between parents and children.

Answer C: Relationship (Opposite Small Individual, Small Individual, Quarter), Difficult. This code does not make clear what the "Quarter" refers to. "Opposite Small Individual" is an appropriate translation of "Parent" but the whole sentence could also be translated as "There are problems at home between parents and children". In any case, the code does not make any reference to the concept of "often".

Answer D: Opposite Seldom, Difficult Situation (Plural Parent, Small Individual). This suggests disputes between parents and children, not the school.

Answer E: (Thought, Quarter), Opposite Seldom, Difficult Relationship, Plural Parent. This code translates the concept of "school" by "Thought Quarter", which could work, particularly since the rest of the code also makes sense. However, the main difference between Answer A and Answer E is that Answer E implies that one group has a difficult relationship with another (e.g. the school has a difficult relationship with the parents), whereas Answer A has an element of reciprocity by placing both parties within the same bracket.

Q1.17 – A: Urgent and E: Decision

Having the word "Mind" would not be of much use since translating the phrase "make up your mind" literally would be difficult using the current code elements. Instead you would be better off translating "make up your mind" as "take a decision". We already have "Take" in the code, so all we need is the word "Decision". This excludes Answer B (Mind) and includes Answer A (Decision)

The word "You" is useless because the phrase does not actually use "you" to point at the reader (as in "you and me") but uses it as "you" = "one", i.e. anyone. This excludes Answer D.

The words "few minutes" can be translated as "Short Time" and retain the same meaning. Answer C is therefore not needed.

The word "Emergency" could be translated by "Increase Difficult Situation", though it would not fully convey the sense of "emergency". As such, the best translation would require a word helping to convey urgency and Answer A is therefore also an option to be retained.

Note the dilemma between Answer A and Answer C. In such cases, you must choose the word that would be the most useful, i.e. adds the most value. In this case, "few minutes" can be translated without the word "minute" without losing too much of its meaning, whereas the concept of "emergency" is central to the sentence and therefore must be conveyed more accurately.

Q1.18 – A: Sphere and B: Around

The word "Mars" (Answer D) could not really be used to describe the Earth accurately; indeed a combination such as "Opposite Mars" could point to any planet. So Answer D is not really appropriate. The Earth would be best described as the Blue Planet, using σ = Blue and Answer A (Sphere) in the absence of a better word for "planet".

The word "One" (Answer E) would have no value as we already have the word "Individual". At a stretch, the concept of "one year" can be coded as "(Opposite Quarter) Season", i.e. (A16)3 since the opposite of one quarter is four. Therefore we do not necessarily need Answer C either. What we cannot code easily though is the concept of "Around" and therefore we would require this word to help out (Answer B).

Note that here also there is a dilemma between Answer C and Answer B. Ideally we would like to have the word "Year" because the way we can code it is convoluted as it stands. However, there is no alternative way of coding "Around" and therefore this word must take preference

Q1.19 – B: Red and E: Speed

The word "Travel" is not required since we already have the word "Transportation". The word "Anger" can be translated as "Difficult Temper" or "Short Temper". This also means that the word "Bad" is not required. We can therefore translate pretty much the exact meaning of anger and flow using current code words.

Red would be useful as, although we can translate "blood" as "Body Liquid", it is not as specific as it could be. There are also no words in the current code that convey the concept of "speed". We could translate it broadly with "Increase Transportation", although this could equally convey the idea of increased volume rather than speed.

DA2 – PRACTICE CODE 2

Q2.1 – C: Taking narcotics is very harmful

6	= Use
$A\Omega$, 3	= Contrary Good, Substance
$\lambda(4,8)$	= Strong (Health, Detriment)

This translates literally as "Using too much of a bad substance is strongly detrimental to health." Answer C fits this coded message best, with narcotics being one interpretation of "Bad Substance".

Answer A: Taking too much cocaine can deteriorate health
This answer fits the general idea of the message, although the use of "too much" makes it more distant than Answer C. The coded message does not contain any notion of "excess", simply of the substance being bad. In addition, the word "can" implies that this may not always be the case, whereas the message is more definite.

Answer B: Many fake medical remedies are very bad for health
Again, this translation fits the general idea of the coded message, although it introduces the notion of "many", implying that some are not that bad for health. The coded message does not make any distinction.

Answer D: The use of medicine can be very prejudicial to health
This does not convey the notion of "Contrary Good". The term "medicine" is too generic.

Answer E: Taking strong medicines makes me feel ill
There is no notion of "individual" in the code and therefore the "me" in this interpretation is not justified. In addition, the code for "Strong" in the message applies to the detriment and not to the substance.

Q2.2 – B: Some illegal drugs are used lawfully for the purpose of medical treatment

AB = Contrary All
AΣ,3 = Contrary Legal, Substance
Σ,6 = Legal, Use
2(K, 10) = Effect (Less, Illness)

This translates literally as "Some (or no) illegal substances have a legal use in order to reduce illness", which closely matches Answer B. Note the difficulty in translating "Contrary All", which could be understood as meaning "some" or "nothing". In such situations you need to see which options are on offer and use the other elements in the message to draw the correct conclusions.

Answer A: No poison is used legally
This does not use the notion of "Less Illness"

Answer C: Some narcotics are believed to be good for use as medication.
There is no notion of "belief" in the coded message. In addition, the coded message conveys that the use as medication is legal/lawful, as opposed to good, which conveys the idea that they achieve good results instead of simply being allowed.

Answer D: Some poisons are legal
This answer does not convey the notion of "Use" or "Less Illness".

Answer E: Not all legal poisons can be used as medication

This does not contain the notion of "Legal Use". Also "Contrary Legal, Substance" would either be translated as "poisons" (though, arguably, some poisons are legal) or "illegal poisons", neither of which fit this answer.

Q2.3 – B: People catch diseases from insects

C(Dα7)   = Plural (Extreme Small Animal)

AΩ2(1)   = Contrary Good Effect (People)

This could be interpreted literally as "Extremely small animals have a bad effect on people" or "People are negatively affected by extremely small animals". In this question, a few options could be suitable and you must therefore carefully analyse the wording used in the translation to determine which option is the closest match.

Answer A: Many people are scared of small animals

The answer mentions "small animals" whilst the coded message talks about "Extreme Small Animals". The use of the word "scared" suggests that this interpretation has applied the word "extreme" to the word "Effect" rather than to the word "Small".

Answer C: Mosquitoes can infect you with malaria

This is not a bad interpretation as "Extreme Small Animals" could be interpreted as "mosquitoes" but the word "malaria" is very specific whereas Answer B has interpreted the word "effect" more generically. Note that the word "you" is not taken as meaning a specific person, but people generally, so it would not be a factor against Answer C.

Answer D: Owning several pets can be detrimental to health

"Pets" is not specific enough to convey the notion of "Extreme Small Animal", and are more likely to be of a medium size.

Answer E: Small insects can be squashed by humans

The coded message suggests that it is the insects that have an impact on people rather than the other way round. "Squashed" is also a strong word to translate "Contrary Good Effect". Answer B is therefore the closest match.

Q2.4 – A: People can become seriously ill by listening to loud music

11, A5 = Intensity, Contrary Silence
ε2(1,4) = Severe Effect (People, Health)

This can be interpreted literally as: "Noise intensity has a severe effect on people's health", i.e. Answer A is the closest.

Note that Answer A introduces the concept of listening to music, i.e. it implies that it is self-inflicted. The coded message is slightly more generic, implying that it is only exposure to loud music which causes the problem. Answer A is therefore not an exact translation but it is the closest.

Answer B: Too much exposure to noise can deteriorate people's hearing ability. This does not convey the idea of intensity, just the length of exposure. It would be more valued if it were phrased as "exposure to loud noises". Also, it specifies that the impact is on hearing ability whereas the coded message is broader, referring to health in general. Finally, the coded message refers to a severe effect, which is not addressed in this answer.

Answer C: Quiet music can be beneficial to people's health
This is taking the opposite meaning to each part of the code. The fact that loud music affects health does not automatically imply that quiet music is beneficial anyway.

Answer D: Loud noises increase people's deafness
There are two degrees of extrapolation required for this translation: (i) there is no notion of "increase" in the coded message, only of "Effect"; (ii) the coded message refers to impact on health rather than deafness. In addition, deafness is not necessarily a severe effect. Answer A is therefore closer.

Answer E: I feel severely unwell when I hear loud music
This is similar to Answer A, but with personalisation (i.e. use of "I") which is not contained in the coded message. In addition, the code explicitly mentions "People", a concept which is not being used here.

Q2.5 – D: Some obese people see themselves as being only overweight

LB	= Negative All
DΔ,1	= Extreme Big, People
H,13	= Reflective, Look
F,Δ	= Only, Big

This could be literally interpreted as "Some very big people look at themselves being only big". This is closely matching Answer D.

Answer A: Some obese people don't look as overweight as they are
This does not make use of the "Reflective" concept, i.e. looking at oneself. Instead this answer describes how others look upon obese people.

Answer B: Not everyone sees obese people as overweight
The coded message does not contain the notion of "other external people", which this answer does. This answer also ignores the "Reflective" concept.

Answer C: Only overweight people watch their weight
This answer does contain the "Reflective" concept, but does not make use of the "Extreme" code. Also, the coded message does not contain the notion of "Only", which this answer does.

Answer E: Some obese people only fancy other obese people
This introduces the notion of "fancy", whereas the coded messages merely mentions "Look". Also, the final part of the coded message only talks of "Big" and not of "obese people". This sentence contains twice the word "obese" and therefore one would expect the code "DΔ,1 = Extreme Big, People" to appear twice in the code.

Q2.6 – C: Some people find it impossible to accept the disabled

LB1	= Negative All People
D(A,12)	= Extreme (Contrary, Tolerant)
Aη, 1	= Contrary Able, People

This can be literally interpreted as "Some people (or, perhaps, no people) are extremely intolerant towards those who are unable". It matches Answer C.

Answer A: Many disabled people don't tolerate their handicap
In the coded message, those who are not tolerant are people in general, as opposed to disabled people. Those who are not tolerated are also described as people and therefore the word "handicap" by itself is not sufficient. In addition, there is no sense of "reflective" feeling in the message, meaning that those who are intolerant and the object of the intolerance are different entities.

Answer B: People are not very tolerant towards the disabled
The notion of "not very" is not a good match for "Extreme (Contrary Tolerant)". Also, the answer starts with "People" when the code is explicit about "Opposite All". This means that the answer cannot be a generalisation.

Answer D: Intolerant people are unable to deal with others
This answer uses most concepts (except "Extreme") but in the wrong way. It also ignores the concept of "Negative All".

Answer E: Many people are not able to show any intolerance
This does not take account of the concept of "Extreme" and does not use the second "People".

Q2.7 – A: Self-important people often don't like others

1(DH17)   = People (Extreme Reflective Love)
EA17   = Generally Contrary Love
CJ   = Plural Other

This can be interpreted literally as "People with extreme love for themselves generally don't like others". This matches Answer A.

Answer B: People don't tend to like those who are vain.
This uses all the right concepts but the wrong way round.

Answer C: Famous lovers can be arrogant
The code refers to reflective love, and not to the love of others. Also "can be" does not suit the notion of "often". The code also involves not loving others, which does not necessarily match the concept of arrogance.

Answer D: People who enjoy reflecting are not very sociable
Although the first part of the sentence could fit the code, the ending is less compatible. The code uses the concept of "Generally" which is not con-

tained in the answer. Also, not being sociable does not mean that they don't love/like others; more that they don't spend or don't like spending time with others.

Answer E: Self-importance will not bring you love
The code talks about people with extreme self-reflecting love not liking/loving others. The answer refers to them not being loved by others.

Q2.8 – D: Brotherly love is often stronger than friendship

17,14	= Love Siblings
E, AK△	= Generally, Contrary Less Big
17,J1	= Love, Other People

This can be literally interpreted as "Love of siblings is generally greater than love of other people", which makes Answer D a good fit. Note that in Answer D, the term brotherly love is used in its generic sense (i.e. meaning love from both brothers and sisters, i.e. siblings, rather than just brothers).

Answer A: Having brothers and sisters tends to make you love others more easily
The original coded message does not have the concept of "easy". Also this translation only uses once the concept of "Love", which features twice in the message.

Answer B: Brotherly love is not always compatible with friendship
This answer does not convey the notion of "Contrary Less Big". It merely talks about incompatibility.

Answer C: Big brothers generally develop better friendships
This does not contain the notion of "Love Siblings".

Answer E: The more obese siblings generally develop better friendships.
In the message, the phrase "Contrary Less Big" does not relate to the siblings but to the love of other people.

Q2.9 – B: Children with no siblings are selfish

C16(L14)	= Plural Child (Negative, Siblings)
FH(13, 18)	= Only Reflective (Look, Listen)

This can be literally interpreted as "Children with no siblings only look at and listen to themselves". This is a good match to Answer B. Looking at the alternatives:

Answer A: Children don't listen to their siblings
The "Negative" relates to "Siblings", not to "Listen"; this translation also does not take account of the word "Look".

Answer C: Some children have siblings who can't hear or see
The "Negative" refers to "Siblings", not to either of the verbs. Also, this interpretation is not using the concept of "Reflective".

Answer D: Children with siblings can't hear themselves talk
This interpretation ignores the concept of "Look". Also, in the message, the "Negative" is associated with "Siblings" and not with "Listen".

Answer E: Children with no siblings don't pay attention to what others say or do. The coded message does not mention "others". This interpretation ignores the "Reflective" concept.

Q2.10 – A: Single mothers are strict disciplinarians

AC   = Contrary Plural
$\pi15$ = Feminine, Parent
$(\lambda,\varepsilon)2(16)$ = (Strong, Severe) Effect (Child)

This can be literally interpreted as "A single mother has a strong and severe effect on a child", which seems to fit Answer A. Looking at the alternatives:

Answer B: Children with only one mother are better raised
However daft this answer looks, most of it fits the coded message given. The only problem is that it introduces the concept of "better", which does not quite match the concept of "severity" introduced by the message.

Answer C: Girls are better raised in single-parent families
The code "Feminine" refers to the parent, not to the child.

Answer D: No mother raises her child well
This translates "Contrary Plural Feminine Parent" as "No mother". Assuming this fits the code, we are still left with an ending which deviates too

much from the original message. Similarly to Answer C, having a strong severe effect on a child does not necessarily equate to being raised well. Option A is closer.

Answer E: The presence of a grandmother influences the development of a child. The concept of "Contrary Plural" is not specifically being used here, i.e. the code "Feminine Parent" would be sufficient to translate grandmother. In addition, the end of the answer mentions "development", which is not a strong enough translation of the concept of "Strong Severe Effect".

Q2.11 – D: Animals used in healthcare research suffer

7, 6	= Animal, Use
1, 4	= People, Health
8, 7	= Detriment, Animal

This can be interpreted literally as "Use of animals in people healthcare causes detriment to the animal". This is close to Answer D. Looking at the alternatives:

Answer A: Animal testing for cosmetic reasons cannot be tolerated
This introduces the concept of tolerance when the coded message refers to detriment to the animal instead. Also, the answer mentions "cosmetic reasons" which are not linked to people's health.

Answer B: Animals involved in experiments get hurt
This answer is also a close match but it mentions "experiments" generally when the coded message makes a point of talking about people's health.

Answer C: Vets sometimes harm animals
Vets would be translated by "Animal Health People" so this answer clearly uses the brackets in the wrong order. This answer does not use the concept of "Animal Use".

Answer E: Humans using animals for healthcare research hurt them
This answer is also a close match but presents it from the point of view of humans hurting animals, rather than the use of animals being detrimental to the animals. Answer D is a closer match, with a similar meaning but an order matching the original more closely.

Q2.12 – E: All blind people should use a guide dog

B, L13, 1   = All, Negative Look, People
γ(6, 7)   = Important (Use Animal)

This can literally be interpreted as "All people who look bad/don't look must use an animal". The closest answer is therefore Answer E. Looking at the alternatives:

Answer A: A sizeable number of blind people have dogs
The code refers to "All people", not just a sizeable number. The word "have" is also slightly weak in relation to the coded word "Use".

Answer B: Not everyone can look after pets
The word "pets" could be an interpretation of "Important Animal". This does not make use of "Use" though.

Answer C: Animals are used to not seeing people
This does not use the concept of "Important" and the order is illogical in relation to the order in which the code words are laid out.

Answer D: Blind animals are of no use to people
The words "Negative Look" refer to people and not to animals. This answer also does not convey the concept of "Important".

Q2.13 – D: The side effects of a potent drug are not negligible

λ2, 4, 3   = Strong Effect, Health, Substance
L(Aλ), CJ2   = [Negative (Contrary Strong), Plural Other Effect]

This can be literally interpreted as: "A drug with a strong effect has other effects which are not weak", which matches Answer D. Looking at the alternatives:

Answer A: Strong drugs generally don't have side effects
This introduces the concept of "generally" which does not feature in the original message. Also, drugs is plural here and the double negative "Negative (Contrary Strong)" is more likely to mean that side effects are not weak rather than they are absent.

Answer B: Drugs' side effects should not be ignored
This does not address directly the concept of "Strong", both in relation to the drug and in relation to the side effects.

Answer C: Side effects affect patients substantially
This does not talk about "Strong Effect Health Substance" at all.

Answer E: All strong drugs have side effects
This does not deal with the strength of the side effects, and also presents drugs in the plural.

Q2.14 – A: (ε, π, 9, 6), (D,5)

Answer A: (Severe, Feminine, Alcohol, Use) (Extreme, Silence)
The first bracket is a close match of the phrase "Alcoholism amongst women". The second bracket "Extreme Silence" can easily be interpreted as "Strong Taboo" i.e. something which is not talked about.

Answer B: People, (Negative, Tolerant), (Feminine, Alcohol, Use)
would translate as "People don't tolerate feminine alcoholism".

Answer C: Severe (Plural, Feminine, People), Generally (Alcohol, Use) would translate as "Severe women are often alcoholics".

Answer D: Strong Alcohol, Severe Effect, Feminine People would translate as "Strong alcohol severely affects women".

Answer E: (Alcohol, Use), Detriment, Feminine People would translate as "Alcohol use is detrimental to women".

Q2.15 – D: (CΣ), (Ω2, 1), E(L2, C7)

Answer D translates as (Plural Legal), (Good Effect, People), Generally (Negative Effect, Plural, Animal), which matches the message to code.

Other answers would translate as follows:

Answer A: (Plural Legal) (Good Effect, Plural Animal) Generally (Negative Effect, People). This would translate as "Laws protecting animals are often against the interest of humans", i.e. exactly the opposite of what the message states.

Answer B: (Plural Legal), Effect (Good People), Generally (Negative Effect, Plural Animal). This would translate as "Laws which have an effect on good people go against the interests of animals".

Answer C: (Plural Legal), (Good Effect, Contrary Animal), Generally (Negative Effect, Plural Animal). This answer is similar to Answer D except that People are coded as "non-animal". Other than the fact that it is in the singular, "non-animal" is not as specific as "People"; it could mean vegetable, mineral, etc. Given the choice between Answer C and Answer D, the latter is more appropriate.

Answer E: (Plural Legal), (Good Effect, People), Generally (Good Effect, Plural Animal). This answer states that the laws are good for both people and animals; it is therefore contradicting the message that needs to be coded.

Q2.16 – C: (7,3), (Σ,6)(Ω13)

Answer C translates as (Animal, Substance), (Legal Use) (Good Look), which would match the message that needs to be translated. The other answers translate as follows:

Answer A: Use (Animal, Substance) (Feminine Substance) Legal
This is not a bad translation albeit that it makes a direct link between the notion of "cosmetic" and "feminine", which is not accurate. Answer C is better suited as it is more generic.

Answer B: Use (Good Look, Animal) Legal
This can be translated as "The use of good-looking animals is legal", which is not appropriate.

Answer D: (Legal, Animal) Use (Good Look, Substance)
This can be translated as "Legal animals use cosmetics", which is not appropriate.

Answer E: Use (Animal, Substance) (Good, Look, Use Feminine People) Important. This answer contains the notion of "feminine use" which is too narrow, and of importance, which is not the same as being legal.

Q2.17 – A: Time and C: Different

The words "personal physical appearance" can be translated by "People Look". The only need therefore is in relation to the first part of the sentence. There is nothing in the code which would help code the notion of "change" or "difference". Therefore Answer C is a good candidate.

The other notion that we need to translate is that of "prolonged use". We already have a word for use and one for alcohol. Prolonged use could be coded as "Big Use" or "Strong Use". However, these two phrases would convey more a notion of volume (i.e. for alcoholics) than the notion of time. Therefore having the word "time" would be useful (Answer A).

DA3 – PRACTICE CODE 3

Q3.1 – A: A taxi ride is more comfortable than a bus ride

HE, 1ε   = Travel Bus, Opposite Comfortable
3(HD)   = Compare (Travel Taxi)

This could literally translate as "Bus travel is not comfortable when compared to taxi travel", i.e. Answer A (with the words presented the other way round but retaining the meaning of the phrase). Looking at the alternatives:

Answer B: Business trips are less comfortable by bus than by taxi
The coded message does not contain the notion of "business trip".

Answer C: A taxi ride does not compare to a bus ride
This does not use the code "Comfortable" and the sentence is presented the wrong way round, with the taxi ride being unfavourable, whereas the coded message presented the taxi ride as the better of the two.

Answer D: Business trips are more comfortable by bus than by taxi
The coded message does not contain the notion of "business trip".

Answer E: Taxis are often more comfortable than buses
The coded message does not contain the notion of "often".

Q3.2 – E: I feel sick when I travel in a car

6(BH)   = Circumstance (Car Travel)
8, 9, Ω   = Personal Feeling Sick

This could literally translate as "When travelling in a car, I feel sick", which suits Answer E. Looking at the alternatives:

Answer A: Car travel can make me sick
The coded message does not contain the notion of "can", i.e. of possibility. It is more definite. Answer E is therefore more appropriate.

Answer B: Travelling in a car can make me sick
Same issue as for Answer A.

Answer C: Car travel leads to car sickness
This does not contain the notion of "Personal" conveyed by code "8". It is therefore too generic to be appropriate.

Answer D: Driving makes me feel sick
This introduces the notion of "driving" (i.e. the person who is talking actually being behind the wheel), when the coded message only refers to travelling in a car (i.e. this could include being a passenger). In that regard, Answer E is closer to the code.

Q3.3 – A: For business trips, taking a train is more convenient than taking a coach

(HA, Σ)   = Travel Train, Convenient
3HF   = Compare Travel Coach
6K   = Circumstance Business

This can be literally translated as "Train travel is convenient when compared to coach travel, when on business", which fits Answer A. Looking at the other answers:

Answer B: Coach travel is less convenient than train travel
This does not use the code "Circumstance Business".

Answer C: Travelling on trains in business class is more convenient than taking a coach. This uses the notion of business class when the coded message is more generic with "Circumstance Business". It also allocated the notion of business class only to the trains when the coded message does not.

Answer D: Business coaches find train travel more convenient
In the message, business is a circumstance, not a person. Also, the coded message does not link directly the terms "Business" and "Coach".

Answer E: Conducting business on a train is easier than on a coach
This could be a good answer as it is very close to the coded message. However, the code is explicit about the fact that it is the travel which is convenient, rather than the conducting of any business. If the 2 "H"s were removed from the coded message, then this would be the correct answer.

Q3.4 – B: Taking a series of several buses can be faster than taking one plane

5(2E)   = Combine (Plural Bus)
7,4 α   = Possibility, Increase Fast
3(1,2,C)   = Compare (Opposite, Plural, Plane)

This can be literally interpreted as: "Combining several buses is possibly faster than a single plane" which matches Answer B. Looking at the other options:

Answer A: Several buses travel faster than planes
This answer does not take account of the "Opposite Plural" concept which precedes "Plane". It also ignores the notion of "Possibility".

Answer C: Taking a plane can be faster than taking a bus
This does not take account of the notion of combining buses.

Answer D: Travelling to the airport by bus is possibly the fastest way. The coded message only mentions planes and no building associated with planes (e.g. Code N for outlet). Also, this answer does not deal with the concept of combining buses.

Answer E: It is possible to travel fast by combining bus and plane travel. This answer does use the notion of combining transport modes but applies it to bus and plane, whereas the coded message was clear about several buses and one plane. This answer also fails to take account of the comparison code (3).

Q3.5 – C: It is faster to travel by car than by combining taxi and bus rides

H5(D,E) = Travel Combine (Taxi, Bus)

1α = Opposite Fast

3(HB) = Compare (Travel Car)

This could be translated literally as "Travelling in a combination of taxi and bus is not fast compared to travelling by car". This suits Answer C, which conveys the same message in a different manner (i.e. by stating that car travel is faster than combining taxi and bus travel). The meaning is unchanged, though. Looking at the alternatives:

Answer A: Travelling by bus or taxi takes longer than by car.
This introduces the notion of choice between bus or taxi, whereas the coded message combines the two.

Answer B: A journey consisting of a taxi ride followed by a bus ride normally takes longer than a car journey. This answer does comply with the requirement to combine taxi and bus, but it imposes an order in the combination (i.e. taxi then bus) which is not included in the coded message. It is therefore more restrictive than Answer C in that regard. In addition, it introduces the concept of "normally", which is also absent from the coded message.

Answer D: It is quicker not to travel by taxi or bus
This does not use the notion of "Car" which the coded message explicitly uses.

Answer E: Travelling by taxi and bus in the same journey is faster than travelling by car. This has the opposite meaning to the coded message.

Q3.6 – E: When I go on holiday, I rent a car

6(1,K) = Circumstance (Opposite, Business)

1, 8, B = Opposite Personal Car

This code is difficult because it is very basic and can be interpreted in many ways. Literally, it can be taken as "When not on business, I use a car that is not mine", which Answer E matches closely. Looking at the alternatives:

Answer A: When business was not going well, I often borrowed a friend's car. This option would be a suitable translation if it were not for the introduction of superfluous concepts such as "not going well" when the coded message simply mentions that it is the opposite of business, and of "often", which does not feature in the code.

Answer B: I use my own car for business purposes
This transforms the double negative (I don't use my own car when not in business) into a positive which is not necessarily correct.

Answer C: I don't have a company car
"I have a company car" could be seen as a translation of "I don't drive my own car", but this would need to be in a business context, whereas the code deals with a non-business context.

Answer D: I never drive alone on business trips
Not driving alone could be an interpretation of not using one's own car. However, the mention of "business trips" makes the answer inappropriate since the circumstance has to be the opposite of business.

Q3.7 – D: There are always several buses travelling together

2E = Plural Bus
λH5(2E) = Always Travel Combine (Plural Bus)

Literally this can be translated as "Several buses always travel with several buses", which matches Answer D closely. Looking at the alternatives:

Answer A: Group travel is best done by bus
The coded message does not contain any notion of "best" or "people".

Answer B: I tend to combine several bus journeys when I travel
The coded message does not contain any notion of "I".

Answer C: Several buses often come at once
This would be a good interpretation of the coded message, if it had "always" instead of "often".

Answer E: Travelling together by bus can be fun
There is no concept of "fun" in the coded message.

Q3.8 – D: Cheap cruises are fast and convenient but not always comfortable

γ(HL,1K) = Cheap (Travel Boat, Opposite Business)

5(α, Σ) = Combine (Fast, Convenient)

1$\lambda\varepsilon$ = Opposite Always Comfortable

This can be interpreted literally as "Boat travel when not on business is both fast and convenient, but not always comfortable", which is close to Answer D. Looking at the alternatives:

Answer A: Cruises are sometimes cheap, fast and convenient but not always comfortable. In the coded message, the code for Cheap is attached directly to the boat travelling and is not part of the bracket which combines fast and convenient. The coded message talks about cheap cruises and not about cruises being cheap.

Answer B: Pleasure boat trips are sometimes cheap, fast and convenient but are rarely comfortable. The error is the same as in Answer A, with the word "cheap" being directly attached to the boat trip rather than part of the combined bracket. In addition, the coded message does not contain the notion of "rarely", only of "not always".

Answer C: Cheap yachts can be fast and convenient but are never comfortable. Most of this answer is appropriate for the coded message given. However, this is talking about cheap yachts rather than cheap boat travel. In the coded message, it is the travelling that is cheap rather than the boat itself.

Answer E: I don't often travel on cheap boats for business purposes as they are often uncomfortable. This answer ignores the notions of "Fast" and "Convenient". Also, the coded message does not contain any notion of "I", which would be typically coded with code 8 = "Personal".

Q3.9 – A: Buying a season ticket is not always cheaper than buying several tickets

5, 2, M   = Combine Plural Ticket
1λ   = Opposite Always
4γ   = Increase Cheap
3, 2, M   = Compare Plural Ticket

This can be literally translated as: "The combination of several tickets is not always cheaper when compared to several tickets", which matches Answer A (with a combination of several tickets being translated as a season ticket). Looking at the alternatives:

Answer B: Buying one return ticket is sometimes cheaper than buying two single tickets. This answer is actually a good fit for the coded message too, but it is too specific. The coded message mentions "Plural" on two occasions, whereas this answer is specific about the number 2. Answer A better reflects the generality of the message.

Answer C: The price of season tickets does not always increase by more than the price of individual tickets. This answer is too complex for the coded message given. The coded message simply compares the price of two alternatives, whereas this translation compares the percentage increase in price.

Answer D: Discounts are often available for those who travel in groups. The word "often" is not a good translation for "not always". Also "Combine Plural Tickets" refers to the purchase of several tickets, which is not necessarily linked to people. "Travelling in groups" refers to people whilst the code refers to tickets.

Answer E: Large families travel more cheaply than individuals
This answer makes no reference to tickets. Also, there is no reference to "Opposite Always" either through "sometimes" or "never".

Q3.10 – B: It can be cheaper and more efficient to purchase a fly-drive ticket from a travel agency

HM5(C,B)   = Travel Ticket Combine (Plane, Car)
7, 4, γ, Δ   = Possibility Increase, Cheap, Efficient

6(KHN) = Circumstance (Business, Travel, Outlet)

This can be literally interpreted as: "A travel ticket combining plane and car is possibly cheaper and more efficient in the circumstance of business travel outlet", which seems to closely match Answer B. Looking at the alternatives:

Answer A: Combined flight-car tickets are often cheaper
This does not make use of the notions of "Efficient" or "Outlet". Also, the word "often" is not an appropriate translation for "Possibility".

Answer C: Organised tours are possibly cheaper than individual trips. The coded message does not contain the notion of "Individual trips". Also this translation does not use "Efficiency".

Answer D: Travel agencies can offer better deals on fly-drive holidays. This does not use the notion of "Efficiency", only of cost.

Answer E: I prefer to buy my cheap fly-drive tickets from the more organised travel agencies. The coded message does not contain the notion of "I". This translation also ignores "Efficient" and introduces the concept of "organised" which is not in the original coded message.

Q3.11 – C: I am starting to feel that my local train station is unsafe

8, π, 9 = Personal, New, Feeling
8AMN = Personal Train Ticket Outlet
1β = Opposite Safe

This can be literally translated as "I have a new feeling that my train ticket outlet is unsafe", which matches Answer C. Looking at the other options:

Answer A: I think that the train station they built recently is unsafe
The coded message associates the word "New" to the word "Feeling" and not to the train station. This answer is therefore inappropriate.

Answer B: I was recently assaulted at my local train station
There is nothing in the coded message about being assaulted, only about the station being unsafe.

Answer D: Local trains have recently been reported as unsafe
This does not use the word "Personal" which the coded message uses twice.

Answer E: I have always felt unsafe at my local train station
The code does not contain the notion of "Always" and in fact makes a point of stating that it is a new feeling.

Q3.12 – D: 1, 2 , 6H, 7, 5(2M)

Answer D translates as "Opposite Plural Circumstance Travel, Possibility, Combine (Plural Tickets) which addresses all the components required to translate the message. Looking at the alternatives:

Answer A: Opposite, Plural, Circumstance Travel, Always Plural Ticket. This answer uses the code for "Always" which is not compatible with "Sometimes".

Answer B: Personal, Travel, Plural, Ticket
This answer uses code "8" for "Personal", which is not contained in the message that needs to be coded.

Answer C: Plural, Circumstance Travel, Opposite Possibility, Plural Ticket. This answer translates as "It is not possible to obtain several tickets for several trips."

Answer E: Possibility (Opposite, Plural, Ticket), Circumstance (Plural Travel). This answer refers to one ticket for several journeys whereas the message mentions one journey with several tickets.

Q3.13 – A: 6(EH), 8, 4(9Ω), 3, 6(LH)

Answer A translates as "Circumstance (Bus Travel), Personal, Increase (Feeling Sick), Compare Circumstance (Boat Travel), which is close to the message that we are trying to code. Looking at the alternatives:

Answer B: Circumstance (Bus Travel) Increase, Sick, Compare, Circumstance Boat. This answer does not code the "I". Also, the last part of the code is "circumstance Boat" as opposed to "Circumstance Boat Travel", so strictly speaking it conveys the message that it is <u>being</u> in a boat rather than <u>travelling</u> in a boat which makes the person feel sick. This translation is therefore not as accurate as Answer A.

Answer C: (Personal, Always, Feeling, Sick), Travel, Compare (Bus Boat). This answer uses the code for "Always" which is not conveyed in the message to code. Also it does not make it clear which mode of transport is making the person sickest.

Answer D: Circumstance (Coach Travel), Personal, Increase, Comfortable, Compare, Circumstance (Boat Travel). This answer uses the notion of "coach" rather than "bus". Also it uses "Comfortable" instead of "Sick".

Answer E: Personal (Feeling, Sick) Circumstance (Bus Travel) Compare Boat. This could translate as I feel sick when I travel by bus, compared to when I am on a boat. This suggests that the person is not necessarily sick in a boat. We would need the notion of "Increase" to make it work, which option A has.

Q3.14 – E: (2, 8), (9, P), 6(HL)

Answer E translates as Plural Personal, Feeling Happiness, Circumstance (Travel Boat), which is close to the message that needs coding. Looking at the alternatives:

Answer A: (Plural, Personal), (Opposite, Feeling, Happiness), Circumstance (Travel Boat). This can be translated as "My friends (or we) don't like sailing" which is the opposite of what the message is saying.

Answer B: (Plural, Personal), (Feeling Happiness), Plural Boat
This answer does address the right concepts though it is not clear as to whether the friends like boats or like sailing. It needs to include the notion of "travel". Answer E is more explicit in that regard.

Answer C: (Plural Personal), (Always, Safe, Feeling), Circumstance (Boat Travel). This translates as "My friends (or we) always feel safe when travelling by boat". This does not contain the notion of "liking" sailing.

Answer D: (Plural Personal), Always Travel Boat

This translates as "My friends always travel by boat" and does not use the notion of "liking".

Q3.15 – B: Late & E: Time

The word "get" can be coded using "Acquire" and therefore we don't need Answers A and D, which in any case imply a payment whilst the word "get" only implies that one is taking possession.

The word "Can" is covered by "Possibility".

This therefore leaves us with "Late" and "Time" which we can combine to code the phrase "At the last minute".

Q3.16 – A: Territory & E: Health

The word "Dangerous" is not needed because we already have "Safe" and we can therefore code "dangerous" as "Opposite Safe".

The word "Trip" is not required because we already have the word "Travel".

This leaves us with "Territory", "Other" and "Health".

The word "Territory" is definitely needed so that we can code "abroad" as "Opposite Personal Territory", which also means that the word "Other" is not required as it is equivalent to "Opposite Personal".

The word "Health" has a relationship with the word "Sick", but "Sick" cannot be used on its own or with any of the current code words to represent the general meaning of "Health". Having "Health" in the code would therefore be more useful.

Q3.17 – A: Build & B: Anger

The word "Makes" is unnecessary because we can use the code for "Feeling".

There is no word in the code which conveys the sense of anger. The word "Sick" is a bit too strong and conveys a different notion, whilst the words

"Opposite Comfortable" are too weak. We would therefore benefit from the word "Anger".

The word "Runway" can be translated by "Plane Road" and therefore the words "Airport and "Runway" are not necessary.

The only word in the code which would convey the notion of "Build" is the word "Acquire", but this implies a purchase or a gift, rather than the action of building, so the word "Build" would also be useful.

DA4 – PRACTICE CODE 4

Q4.1 – C: Heavy holiday departures cause traffic jams

3, 16   = Large, Departure
E9   = Opposite Work
FE(15,7) = Consequence Opposite (Traffic Fluid)

This can be literally interpreted as "A large departure for the opposite of work has as a consequence non-fluid traffic", which matches Answer C relatively well. Looking at the alternatives:

Answer A: Mass redundancies provoke strikes that cripple the country. This answer interprets each component differently, with:
- Large departure = Mass redundancies
- Opposite Work = Strikes
- Opposite (Traffic Fluid) = Cripple the country.

In this answer the strikes are a consequence and therefore should feature in the code after the F code for "Consequence". Also, the answer introduces the notion of "country" which is not in the original code.

Answer B: Commuters cause traffic congestion
This answer relates to work since it talks of commuters, although it is not clear whether they are arriving or leaving work (the coded message states that we are dealing with departures). The answer also does not make use of "Large".

Answer D: Getting stuck in traffic whilst going on holiday can be stressful. The coded message does not contain anything about stress.

Answer E: Long holidays always involve traffic jams

The coded message does not have the notion of "always". In addition, it contains the notion of "Departure", which this answer does not use (it simply says "involve"). Finally, the word "Large" applies to the departure rather than the duration of the holiday.

Q4.2 – A: Hatred of others sometimes leads to war

10	= Hate
E (B11)	= Opposite (Same Person)
GC	= Negative Always
FA14	= Consequence Amplify Discord

This can be literally interpreted as: "Hating other people sometimes (or not always) leads to greater discord", which matches the meaning of Answer A. Looking at the alternatives:

Answer B: Selfishness sometimes paves the way for conflict

The notion of selfishness has more to do with loving oneself than with hating others. This would work if the code was "Opposite Hate, Same Person". In addition, the word "conflict" is equivalent to the word "Discord" and therefore this answer does not make use of "Amplify".

Answer C: People who hate others never agree with anyone

This answer does not convey the notion of "Consequence" or "Amplify".

Answer D: It's often the same people who are looking for trouble

There is no notion of "Hate" or "Opposite Same People".

Answer E: Most people hate those who look for trouble

There is no concept of "most people" in the coded message. In addition, this answer does not make use of "Negative Always" or "Consequence".

Q4.3 – B: Agricultural decline causes lack of food in cities

(E17), 18	= (Opposite Rise), Farm
F(Eπ, 6)	= Consequence Opposite Full, Food
3, 1	= Large Population

This can be interpreted as "A decline in farm has the consequence of empty food for a large population", which is the message that Answer B is trying to convey. Looking at the alternatives:

Answer A: Smaller farms produce better food for customers
This does not use the notion of "Rise". Also the coded message does not introduce any kind of comparison on quality, or the idea of customers. The concept of "Large Population" cannot be extrapolated to mean "customers" as easily as it can be extrapolated to mean "city".

Answer C: Poor harvesting provoked starvation for the whole population. This is not a bad translation, except that it talks in the past tense, which the coded message does not do. Also, the concept of "whole population" is an exaggeration on the "Large Population" present in the coded message.

Answer D: It takes fewer farmers to produce enough food for cities
This does not contain the notion of "Consequence", i.e. it is not because there are fewer farmers that enough food is produced.

Answer E: The decreasing number of farms is not sufficient to fulfil the increasing need in food in growing cities. This answer ignores the notion of "Consequence". Also the coded message does not contain the notion of "increasing need" or "growing cities".

Q4.4 – A: Brainstorming encourages productivity

5, 2   = Pool, Idea
FA9   = Consequence Amplify Work

This can literally be translated as "Pooling ideas amplifies work", which corresponds to Answer A. Looking at the other answers:

Answer B: I work better at the poolside
This does not use the concept of "Idea".

Answer C: I think better after a good swim
The coded message does not have the concept of "good" associated with "Pool". Also, it is the work that should be amplified, not the thinking/ideas.

Answer D: I have the idea of building a fishpond
This does not use the code "Amplify".

Answer E: Leisure times help people work harder
This does not use the code "Idea".

Q4.5 – E: Low supply leads to the development of a black market

E3, 15   = Opposite Large, Traffic
F, 17   = Consequence, Rise
Eα,15   = Opposite Legal, Traffic

This can be interpreted as "Small traffic leads to a rise in illegal traffic", which is the meaning of Answer E. Looking at the alternatives:

Answer A: There aren't many illegal goods around
This does not convey the fact that there is a rise in illegal traffic.

Answer B: Traffickers control the food market
The code does not mention "food". Also this does not convey the fact that the illegal traffic is a consequence of a lack of supply.

Answer C: It is illegal to close down small markets
This does not convey the concept of "Consequence".

Answer D: It is illegal to drive on market days
This answer does not contain the notion of "Opposite Large" or of "Consequence".

Q4.6 – B: Lack of resources always provokes migration

(E, π)   = Opposite Full
(9, 6)   = Work, Food
CF(1, 4, 16)   = Always Consequence (Population Intense Departure)

This can be literally translated as "Not having full employment and food supplies always leads to intense departure of population", which matches the meaning of Answer B, with the word "resources" encompassing both work and food. Looking at the other answers to check if any are closer:

Answer A: Birds migrate to look for food
This answer narrows the scope down to birds, whereas the original coded message is more generic. In fact, it mentions work, which is unlikely to apply to birds, and as such is ignored in this answer.

Answer C: Displacement of people is often caused by the lack of resources. The use of "displacement" does not reflect the concept of "Intense Departure" in the way that "migration" does, though this is debatable. In any case, the use of the word "often" contradicts the presence of the word "Always" in the coded message.

Answer D: Farm workers always travel a lot to look for work
This answer ignores the concepts of "Opposite Full" and "Intense". This also fails to convey the notion of "Consequence".

Answer E: Most people go shopping at the weekend
This has no notion of "Consequence". Also, the code "Always" is not present in this translation, since it only mentions "Most people".

Q4.7 – A: Slavery will not be abolished

$E\gamma$ (1,9)   = Opposite Free (Population, Work)
$DE(E\alpha)$ = Future Opposite (Opposite Legal)

This can be literally interpreted as "The work population which is not free in future will not be illegal", which matches the message conveyed by Answer A with some degree of interpretation since "will not be illegal" effectively means that it will remain legal and therefore will not be abolished. To be sure that this is the closest answer we can find, we need to check the alternatives:

Answer B: Some prisons will close in the near future
This talks about "some" whereas the coded message is more generic. Also, this answer does not address the issue of "Work" and introduces a concept of "near future" when the coded message is only talking about the future generally. Finally, the coded message contains "not illegal", which is not well translated by "some prisons will close", as this conveys the opposite meaning.

Answer C: Salaried workers are legal
This contains no notion of "Future" and fails to use the notion of "Free".

Answer D: Slavery will be illegal
This ignores the double negative "Opposite (Opposite Legal)", which converts to "not illegal" rather than "illegal".

Answer E: Making prisoners work will no longer be legal
This fails to translate the double negative, i.e. it should be "will no longer be illegal".

Q4.8 – D: More people are coming to do voluntary work on farms

1, γ, 9, 18   = Population, Free, Work, Farm
A15, E16   = Amplify Traffic, Opposite Departure

This can be literally translated as "The population with free work on a farm increases traffic for arrivals", which matches closely the meaning of Answer D. Looking at the alternatives:

Answer A: There are many volunteers on farms
This does not make allowance for "Amplify".

Answer B: Pensioners like visiting farms
This does not make allowance for "Amplify". In addition, the coded message contains no notion of "liking".

Answer C: More and more people leave farming jobs to work elsewhere as volunteers. The coded message is clear about "Opposite Departure", which this answer contradicts.

Answer E: Freelance workers will increasingly be accepted in farming jobs. This answer contains the notion of "future" which the coded message does not contain. Also, freelance workers are independent workers, but not necessarily free.

Q4.9 – C: Road rage will be rewarded by a prison sentence

15, 12   = Traffic Path
3, 14   = Large Discord
DCF(Eγ)   = Future Always Consequence (Opposite Free)

This can be literally translated as "A traffic path large discord will always lead to not being free", which Answer C interprets well. Looking at the alternatives:

Answer A: Those who campaign against road building programmes are likely to be jailed. The coded message does not contain the notion of "likely", otherwise this would be a close runner-up to Answer C. This answer also personalises the problem ("Those who") whereas the coded message talks about the problem more generically which also makes Answer C more suitable.

Answer B: Arguments against road charges are inconsequential
This ignores the "Future". Also the term "inconsequential" would only be valid if "Opposite" applied to "Consequence", which it does not.

Answer D: Severely damaging a road will give rise to a fine
"Damaging a road" is not the same as a "Discord", which implies a disagreement.

Answer E: An argument about travel directions could cost you dear
This ignores the concept of "Large Discord" as it merely mentions an argument,

Q4.10 –A: Tides are slowing down departures

7, β	= Fluid Level
(17, E17)	= Rise, Opposite Rise
FEA, 16, 15	= Consequence Opposite Amplify Departure Traffic

This can be literally interpreted as "The rise and fall of fluid level is reducing departure traffic", which closely matches Answer A. Looking at the other answers:

Answer B: Boats come and go depending on the tide
The "come and go" should apply to the water, not to the boats. This answer ignores the "Opposite Amplify" concept.

Answer C: Boats make waves
This does not convey the notion of "Departure". Also, the waves (or tide) are not the consequence; they are the cause.

Answer D: Owners need to evacuate the water from their boat before departing.
The coded message does not mention anything about people (owners), and time (before departing). In fact, the coded message does not even mention anything about boats.

Answer E: Boats leave port at high tide and not at low tide
The coded message does not have any negativity attached to low tide.

Q4.11 – C: Wealth has no bearing on intelligence

π, 8	= Full Money
EF	= Opposite Consequence
π (3,2)	= Full (Large Idea)

This can be literally translated as "A lot of money has no consequence on a lot of big ideas", which makes Answer C a good contender. Looking at the alternatives:

Answer A: A lot of money can give you an interesting life
This uses "can" and therefore introduces an element of probability which is not contained in the coded message (which is more definite).

Answer B: Wealthy people are not the more tolerant
The link between tolerance and large ideas is tenuous. Also, the coded message does not mention people explicitly and therefore Answer C is closer from that point of view.

Answer D: Creativity brings expenses
This does not allow for the "Opposite Consequence" and in any case sets outs the elements in the wrong order. It should be "Expenses have no impact on creativity".

Answer E: Prosperity sometimes goes with a boring life
"Goes with" is not a sign of consequence, simply of association. Also, "Opposite" applies to "Consequence" and not to "Large Idea".

Q4.12 –B: 8, EC, F(δ, 11)

Answer B translates as "Money, Opposite Always, Consequence (Positive Person) which is close to the original message that we were asked to code. Looking at the other answers:

Answer A: "Money Consequence (Opposite Positive, Person)"
This means "Money makes you unhappy", which is not quite what the original message stated.

Answer C: "Money, Opposite Amplify, Positive, Idea"

This literally means that "Money reduces your happiness". This code also does not convey the notion of "not always".

Answer D: "Rise Money Amplify Intense Positive"

This means "A pay increases makes you feel better". It refers to a rise in money rather than the presence of money. Also, this ignores the "not always" notion.

Answer E: "(Negative Pool Money) Opposite Amplify, Positive Person".

This which means very little, though suggests that the person is getting depressed as a result of debts.

Q4.13 – C: Probability

Optimist can be coded with δ, 2, 11 = "Positive Idea Person".
Pay rise can be coded with 8, 17 = "Money Rise".
Increase is not needed since we already have "Rise".
Happy would only be needed to code "Optimist" which we can do in other ways, as shown above.

The phrase "better chance" would require the notion of probability, which is difficult to code based on current code words. This is therefore the correct answer.

Q4.14 – C: Stone & E: Live

"Few" can be coded as $E3\beta$ = "Opposite Large Level".
"High" can be coded as "Large Level".
"Tribe" can be coded as "Pool Person" or "Pool Population".

There is nothing in the code, however, to help translate "rocky" and therefore Answer C (Stone) is needed. Similarly the notion of "live" can only be translated very indirectly by using "Work and Farm" and therefore would be useful too (Answer E).

DA5 – PRACTICE CODE 5

Q5.1 – D: As the conductor moves his baton, the orchestra starts playing

1(10, 16) = Master (Shift, Stick)
F   = Consequence
AC, 12, 7 = Opposite Singular, Instrument, Start

This can be literally translated as "The master shifting the stick has the consequence that several instruments start", which fits Answer D well. Looking at the alternatives:

Answer A: The karate master starts teaching traditional weapons
This answer does not convey the notion of "Consequence" and introduces the concept of "traditional", which is not contained in the coded message.

Answer B: The experienced boatman starts rowing with two paddles
This does not contain the notion of "Consequence".

Answer C: The commander is at the helm and is shouting orders to start lowering the sails
The coded message mentions a stick of some sort, which is not used in this translation. The coded message also does not contain any notion of "shouting" or "lowering". Finally, translating "instrument" into "sails" is far-fetched.

Answer E: The shepherd can play several instruments
The notion of "Stick" is conveyed only implicitly through the word "shepherd" and the message does not convey the notion of "Consequence" or "Start".

Q5.2 – E: The museum used to present good exhibitions

2, 11   = Art, Building
(AC)(Σ13)= Opposite Singular (Good Show)
D14   = Past Period

This can be literally interpreted as "The art building had good shows in the past", which matches Answer E well. Looking at the alternatives:

Answer A: It is interesting to show how this piece of art was made
This does not make use of "Building" or "Opposite Singular".

Answer B: This art gallery never displayed any nice paintings
Never is a bad translation of "Opposite Singular", which really means "Several".

Answer C: Architecture from antiquity can be seen in many sites
This does not use the notion of "Good".

Answer D: Every year, I visited a museum and saw nice exhibitions
The coded message does not contain the notion of "I". It also does not mention any regular visiting (only the past). This answer is not "bad", but Answer E is closer.

Q5.3 – A: The marble sculpture can't be removed; it's too heavy!

Ω, 15	= Over, Weight
F	= Consequence
AE	= Opposite Possibility
10, 8, 2	= Shift Stone Art

This can be literally translated by "Excess weight means that this stone art cannot be shifted" or "He is obese and therefore cannot move this stone art". Answer A is close to the first interpretation. Looking at the alternatives:

Answer B: I ate too much; I can't visit another monument
The coded message mentions being overweight rather than having eaten too much, though this could be an acceptable translation. This translation contains a notion of "past" which is not included in the coded message. More importantly, this translation ignores the notion of "Shift", translating it badly as "visiting", and contains the notion of "I" which is not included in the original message.

Answer C: This heavy obelisk is impossible to displace
All the right concepts are included within this interpretation, except the notion of "Consequence". Indeed, this translation does not mean that it is the weight of the obelisk which makes it difficult to displace, simply that it is a heavy obelisk which is difficult to move.

Answer D: Removing a big piece of jewellery is quite impossible
This does not convey the notion of "Overweight" or "Consequence".

Answer E: I can't take it upon myself to get rid of this sculpture
This interpretation has the notion of "I", which is not included in the original message. It also ignores the concept of "Overweight".

Q5.4 – B: The violin player will soon be a soloist

4, 9, 12   = Person, Wood, Instrument
ΔAD   = Near Opposite Past
C1   = Singular Master

This can be literally interpreted as "The person with wood instrument will be a single master in the close future", which matches Answer B. Looking at the alternatives:

Answer A: The woodcutter is my neighbour's only teacher
The codeword "Near" applies to "Opposite Past", not to a person, hence it can't be used to mean "neighbour". In addition, this interpretation does not contain the notion of "Opposite Past", i.e. future.

Answer C: This string instrument maker will one day make a masterpiece. The coded message does not contain the notion of "string", only of "Wood". In addition, the concept of "near" cannot be translated by "one day", which implies something more distant.

Answer D: In the future, craftsmen will work with natural materials
In the coded message, the concept of "Wood" is used to qualify the person, not a working material. This answer also ignores the concept of "Singular".

Answer E: This harpist is a promising student
This answer makes too many assumptions. The "harp" is a very loose translation for "Wood Instrument". In addition, the word "promising" implies a notion of future, but the coded message is more definite, implying that it will happen rather than it might happen. The term "promising" would be translated by "Opposite Past, Possibility".

Q5.5 – A: During the Stone Age, many weapons' handles were made of wood

8, 14	= Stone, Period
AC12	= Opposite Singular Instrument
9, 16	= Wood Stick

This can be literally interpreted as "In the stone period, there was more than one instrument with a wood stick", which is close to Answer A. Looking at the alternatives:

Answer B: Diamond trade was organised by canoe
This does not make use of the "Opposite Singular Instrument". Also the translation of "Wood Stick" into canoe is tenuous.

Answer C: During the gold rush, people would make their own tools with wood. This does not use the notion of "Stick".

Answer D: When you are stoned, you can feel a bit wooden
The connection between "Stone Period" and "stoned" is dubious. Also, this does not take account of "Opposite Singular" or "Stick".

Answer E: Several instruments, such as recorders, are made of wood. This does not use the concept of "Stone Period".

Q5.6 –A: Excessive urbanisation can lead to deforestation

Ω11	= Over Building
EF	= Possibility Consequence
AB9	= Opposite Increase Wood

This can be literally interpreted as "Building too much might lead to a decrease in wood", which is close to Answer A. However, there are several other close possibilities. Looking at the alternatives:

Answer B: Building too many houses means too much wood is used
This answer is also close, except that it does not use the "Possibility" as it is more definite. Also, it says that too much wood is being used whereas the code mentions an "Opposite Increase". This is ambiguous because one could argue that too much wood being used means a decrease in wood supply, but this requires too much extrapolation.

Answer C: Wood is used less and less to build skyscrapers
This does not convey the concept of "Consequence" or "Possibility".

Answer D: Scaffoldings can be made of wood
This does not convey the concept of "Consequence".

Answer E: From the roof, we can hardly see a tree
The word "Opposite" is not applied to "Possibility" in the coded message.

Q5.7 –C: An archaeologist looks at old cemeteries and old cities

1, 6, D	= Master, Save, Past
5	= Look
AC	= Opposite Singular
D, 4, 8	= Past Person Stone
D, 4, 11	= Past Person Building

This can literally be interpreted as "A master at saving the past looks at several stones associated with past people and several buildings associated with past people", which matches Answer C well. Looking at the alternatives:

Answer A: My teacher checked if we brought dangerous objects in
The word "teacher" does not convey the notion of "Save Past". Instead this translation used the word "Past" to mean the past tense. This sentence also does not make any reference to "Person", "Stone", or "Building".

Answer B: Ancient medicine men used stones and buildings inherited from their ancestors. This does not use the notion of "Look".

Answer D: The first bankers believed in investing in ancient stones and ancient buildings. This does not use the notion of "Look". Also the word "first" is not contained in the original coded message, nor can it be derived easily from anything in the coded message.

Answer E: My first clock was taken from an old building and looked like it was made of stone. The coded message does not have the notion of "clock" or anything relating to keeping the time. Also, in the message, "Past Person Stone" and "Past Person Building" are on a par footing. In this sentence, they are not.

Q5.8 –B: A projector makes an artist look better

17, 12   = Light, Instrument
BΣ5   = Increase Good Look
13, 1   = Show, Master

This can be literally translated as "A light instrument increases the good look for a show master", which matches Answer B closely. Looking at the alternatives:

Answer A: The gadget demonstrator convinces others that his product is the best. The coded message talks about "Increase Good Look", i.e. improving the image, whereas this translation talks about "convincing that the product is the best". There is of course a relationship, but it requires more extrapolation than Answer B. Also, in the code, "Light Instrument" and "Show Master" are separated, whereas in this translation they are put together to code "gadget demonstrator".

Answer C: The lighthouse helps boatmen see better
This does not use the notion of "Show". The word "boatmen" is also in the plural whilst, in the coded message, the word "Master" is in the singular. In addition, the word "boatmen" is not strong enough to translate "Master". We would require at least "Experienced boatmen", or something of that order.

Answer D: Fireworks are more and more beautiful
This does not use the word "Master".

Answer E: The clown uses a mirror that makes people look good
This does not use "Increase".

Q5.9 – E: The captain scans the sea for a possible dangerous rock

1(18, 11) = Master (Water, Building)
5, 18   = Look Water
E(Aπ8)   = Possibility (Opposite Safe Stone)

This can literally translate into "The master of the water building looks at the water for a possible unsafe stone", which closely matches Answer E. Looking at the alternatives:

Answer A: The water tower's manager dropped stones into the water
The coded message uses the code for "Look", which bears no relation to "dropped". Also the message is not in the past tense, whereas this translation is. Finally, this answer does not make use of "Opposite Safe".

Answer B: I see water falling dangerously from the dam onto rocks
The code does not talk about water falling. Also, the notion of "Opposite Safe" should apply to the rocks and the coded message does not contain the notion of "I".

Answer C: An experienced diver scans the sea for dangerous rocks
This does not use the notion of "Building", it has "rocks" in the plural and ignores "Possibility".

Answer D: The dangerous mountain is visible from the huge bridge across the bay. This is a very convoluted translation. The code "Master (Water Building)" could, at a stretch, mean "bridge". "Opposite Safe Stone" could mean "dangerous mountain across", but the terms need to be arranged in a very different order in order for this answer to work. For example, across the bay is really a translation of "Opposite Water". In addition, this answer does not use the notion of "Possibility".

Q5.10 – A: Too much water pressure may endanger people

(18, 15) Ω= (Water, Weight) Over

E   = Possibility

A (π, 4)   = Opposite (Safe, Person)

This can be literally translated as "Excess of water weight can make the opposite of a safe person", which is similar to Answer A (with an interpretation needed to translate water weight into "water pressure"). Looking at the alternatives:

Answer B: Drinking too much water may be a cause of obesity
This uses the word "Weight" twice (once for "too much water" and once for "obesity").

Answer C: Giving too much water to a dehydrated person can be dangerous. The coded message does not mention anything about a "dehydrated person".

Answer D: It is impossible to transport water to a drought-suffering nation. This does not make use of "Possibility" and contains a notion of "drought" which is not present in the original coded message.

Answer E: One should be careful when carrying water
This does not use the notion of "Weight" and "Over". Being careful also does not necessarily mean that it is unsafe.

Q5.11 – B: Always & E: Outside

The word "Risk" is not required since we already have the word "Safe".
The word "Lightning" is not required since we already have "Light".
The word "Swimming" can be translated by "Water Building".
The word "during" can be translated with "Period".
The phrase "open-air" is more difficult to translate with the current code without naming everything that can be found outside. Therefore, a code for "Outside" would be useful (Answer E).

Finally, the word "Never" cannot easily be translated using the current code and the addition of the word "Always" (Answer B) would allow to translate is as "Opposite Always".

MOCK

EXAM

MOCK EXAM INSTRUCTIONS

Over the following pages, you will find a full mock exam for the UKCAT. This contains the required number of questions for each of the main four sections.

At the beginning of each section, we have indicated the number of questions included and the maximum amount of time that you can spend on each section. The time shown is the time that you can spend on answering questions (i.e. it does not include the 1-minute administration time that you will be given on the day of the test to read some basic instructions.

You should allow 1 hour and 26 minutes in total for this mock exam, to be allocated as follows:

- Page 289: Quantitative Reasoning: 21 minutes
- Page 307: Abstract Reasoning: 15 minutes
- Page 321: Verbal Reasoning: 21 minutes
- Page 345: Decision Analysis: 29 minutes

You will be reminded of these timings at the start of each section. When the time allotted to one section has expired, you must move on to the next section (i.e. you cannot use left-over time from one section to spend more time on another).

For the purpose of the quantitative reasoning questions, you are allowed a hand-held calculator.

Note: the actual UKCAT has an additional 4 minutes for administration purposes (1 minute per section) + an additional 30 minutes for the fifth part of the test (Non-cognitive analysis), making a total of 2 hours. However since there is no value in preparing for the latter and that it is ignored for the purpose of selection for entry into medical school, we have excluded it from this mock exam.

Once you have taken the full mock exam, use the marking schedule on page 409 to calculate your score.

MOCK EXAM

QUANTITATIVE REASONING

(10 sets of 4 questions – 21 minutes)

QR 1/10
Mock
Bottling It Up

A mail order wine company sells wines either as individual bottles or in cases of 12 bottles.

The prices, in pounds, are set out in the table below:

Wines	Case of 12 bottles on or after 01/01/08	Case of 12 bottles on or after 01/01/09	Case of 12 bottles on or after 01/01/10	Per bottle on or after 01/01/09
Red Gold Medal Winner 2007	57	40	49	6.67
White Gold Medal Winner 2007	52	39	44	6.50
White mixed case	36	24	40	4
Red mixed case	43	33	37	5.50
Classic White Selection	48	36	39	6
Classic Red Selection	50	33	25	4.40

MOCK EXAM QUESTIONS

Q1.1 By what percentage was the case of 12 bottles of White Gold Medal Winner 2007 discounted between 2008 and 2009?

a. 13%   **b.** 15%   **c.** 17%   **d.** 25%   **e.** 33%

Q1.2 On Christmas Eve 2009, a customer wishes to purchase one case of each type. He has a voucher granting an 11% discount on all white wines and 13% discount on all red wines. What is the total cost?

a. £180.33   **b.** £180.47   **c.** £181.11   **d.** £191.11   **e.** £193.04

Q1.3 In June 2009, a customer wants to buy one case of wine. Out of the five following options, he wishes to choose the one which offers the biggest saving in pounds between purchasing one case and purchasing individual bottles. Which option should he choose?

Option 1: White Gold Medal Winner 2007
Option 2: White mixed case
Option 3: Red mixed case
Option 4: Classic White Selection
Option 5: Classic Red Selection

a. Option 1   **b.** Option 2   **c.** Option 3   **d.** Option 4   **e.** Option 5

Q1.4 In June 2009, a customer wishes to purchase wines from the Classic Red Selection. How much does the customer save by buying a case rather than 12 individual bottles, expressed as a fraction of the total "per bottle" cost?

a. 3/8   **b.** 2/7   **c.** 4/7   **d.** 4/9   **e.** 2/3

QR 2/10
Mock

Waste Management

Average waste per individual for 1982 (in kg)

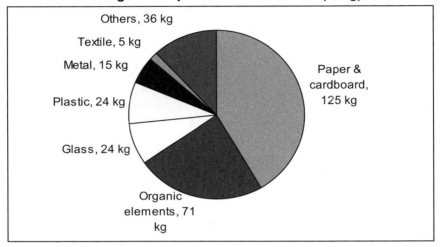

Average waste per individual for 1992 (in kg)

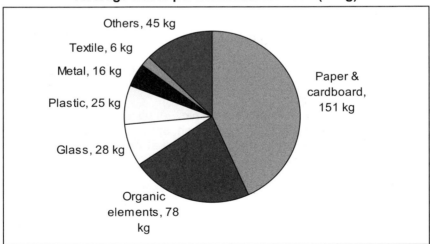

Profile of waste per individual for 2002
(as a % of total weight of individual waste)

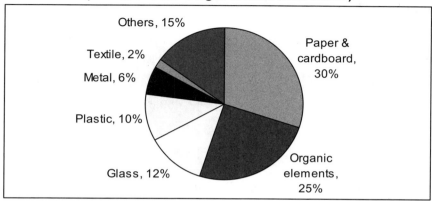

In 2002, the average weight of glass thrown away by inhabitants of Greentown was 54kg. In that year, Greentown, a town with 8700 inhabitants, recycled: 57.31% of cardboard and paper, 80% of organic elements, 80% of glass, 22% of plastic, 80% of metal, 40% of textile and 5% of everything else.

MOCK EXAM QUESTIONS

Q2.1 What was the average total weight of waste per individual in 2002?

    a. 250kg   **b.** 300kg   **c.** 350kg   **d.** 400kg   **e.** 450kg

Q2.2 By how much in percentage did the weight of paper and cardboard waste increase between 1982 and 1992?

    a. 8.0%   **b.** 10.6%   **c.** 14.7%   **d.** 20.8%   **e.** 21.2%

Q2.3 In 2002, what percentage of the total recycled weight did recycled textile represent?

    a. 0.15%   **b.** 1.15%   **c.** 1.45%   **d.** 2.10%   **e.** 2.26%

Q2.4 How many kilos of organic elements were not recycled in 2002?

    a. 193,720   **b.** 195,750   **c.** 206,240   **d.** 213,230   **e.** 783,000

QR 3/10 Mock   The Big Freeze

Equivalence between different temperature scales

Unit of temperature	Formula
Kelvin [K]	= ([°F] + 459.67) x 5/9
Rankine [R]	= 9/5 x [K]
Celsius [°C]	= ([°F] − 32) x 5/9

Where [°F] = Fahrenheit

MOCK EXAM QUESTIONS

Q3.1 Two international explorers look at their own thermometers. One is graduated in Fahrenheit, the other in Celsius but they both show the same number. What is this number?

  a. − 50   **b.** − 48   **c.** − 40   **d.** − 36   **e.** − 32

Q3.2 Water boils at 100 °C. What is this temperature in Rankine?

  a. 355.37   **b.** 373.15   **c.** 396.27   **d.** 574.26   **e.** 671.67

Q3.3 The average temperature of the human body is 309.95 Kelvin. What is this temperature in Fahrenheit?

  a. 97.97   **b.** 98.24   **c.** 98.34   **d.** 98.56   **e.** 98.60

Q3.4 Currently, the average temperature of the Earth's surface is 15 °C. With warming, scientists expect a rise of the average Celsius temperature by 16% over the next century. What will be the average Earth surface temperature in the next century, expressed in Fahrenheit?

  a. 63.21   **b.** 63.32   **c.** 65.36   **d.** 66.58   **e.** 68.44

QR 4/10 Mock	Running Wild

MOCK EXAM QUESTIONS

Q4.1 A mother rabbit and her son Skippy are at the same point in a field, preparing to move forward in the same linear direction. At 8am, Skippy moves forward at a speed of 1.2 km/h. His mother remains motionless until 8.16am, at which point Skippy stops and his mother decides to catch up with him, moving at a speed of 2.4 km/h. How long will it take for her to catch up with him?

a. 4 mins   **b.** 8 mins   **c.** 16 mins   **d.** 24 mins   **e.** 32 mins

Q4.2 Skippy and his mother are both jumping clockwise along the perimeter of the field (33m long). In one second, Skippy jumps a ground distance of 20cm whilst his mother jumps a ground distance of 50cm. After 25 seconds, Skippy gets tired and stops. He remains still, waiting for his mother to catch up with him. From that moment on, how many seconds will it take his mother to reach him, assuming she carries on jumping on his clockwise circuit along the field perimeter at the same speed?

a. 24s   **b.** 38s   **c.** 41s   **d.** 51s   **e.** 76s

Q4.3 When Father rabbit hops on his right foot, he moves forward by 20cm. When he hops on his left foot, he moves forward by 40cm. When he jumps on both feet he moves forward by 70cm. What is the minimum number of jumps he must do in order to travel exactly 198m?

a. 280   **b.** 282   **c.** 284   **d.** 286   **e.** 288

Q4.4 Father rabbit is at point A and Mother rabbit is at point B, 1500m away. They want to meet up and start their journey at the same time, travelling in a straight line. It normally takes the father 20 minutes to travel the whole distance. The mother's speed is 7/9 of the father's. At which distance from point B will they meet?

a. 656.25m   **b.** 843.75m   **c.** 966.75m   **d.** 1,057.66m **e.** 1166.66m

QR 5/10 Mock

Fruit Harvest

Years	Apricots Category A		Apricots Category B	
	Production (in tons)	Sales price per kg	Production (in tons)	Sales price per kg
2002	404	£ 0.75	300	£ 0.85
2003	73	£ 1.05	52	£ 1.20
2004	513	£ 0.60	354	£ 0.75
2005	417	£ 0.70	312	£ 0.80
2006	114	£ 0.95	57	£ 1.15

Years	Nectarines Category C		Nectarines Category D	
	Production (in tons)	Sales price per kg	Production (in tons)	Sales price per kg
2002	113	£ 0.95	80	£ 1.05
2003	64	£ 1.15	35	£ 1.25
2004	132	£ 0.85	97	£ 1.00
2005	120	£ 0.80	87	£ 1.15
2006	72	£ 1.10	37	£ 1.30

Note: 1 ton = 1,000kg

MOCK EXAM QUESTIONS

Q5.1   In which year was the total income from the sale of Apricots Category A the highest?

a. 2002   **b.** 2003   **c.** 2004   **d.** 2005   **e.** 2006

Q5.2   Which category brought the highest income over the period covering 2002–2006?

a. Apricots Category A   **b.** Apricots Category B
c. Nectarines Category C   **d.** Nectarines Category D

Q5.3   In 2003, a hailstorm destroyed most of the production. Had the fruit grower installed anti-hail nets on his orchard, his production would have increased by 40% in each of the four categories but prices would have remained at the same level.

We know that:

▶   His orchard contains 110 rows of trees, each 654 feet long.
▶   An anti-hail net covers 2 rows.
▶   An anti-hail net costs £3 per foot.

Had he installed the net in 2003, what would his profit have been?

a. £ 143,140 **b.** £ 251,050 **c.** £ 300,438 **d.** £ 358,960 **e.** £ 466,870

Q5.4   Apricot nectar is a drink made by crushing apricots and extracting the juice and pulp. Nothing else is added. We know that:

▶   Category A apricots produce 65% of their weight in nectar
▶   Category B apricots produce 72% of their weight in nectar
▶   1 litre of apricot nectar weighs 1.2kg

How many litres of nectar will be produced by using the entire 2006 apricot production?

a. 95,950   **b.** 115,140   **c.** 138,168   **d.** 176,535   **e.** 189,732

QR 6/10 Mock	Sweet Music

Six villages with a total population of 10,276 inhabitants got together in 2004 to create a school for music and dance. The overall population does not change from year to year.

In 2005, the school spent £58,650.

In 2006, the total expenditure increased by 2.7%. In that year, Violintown and Drumtown, the two most populated villages, shared equally half of the new amount. The other villages shared the rest of the charges in proportion to the number of pupils each village had in the school in 2006.

Villages	Number of pupils 2005	Number of pupils 2006
Clarinetown	43	38
Drumtown	65	56
Flutetown	11	10
Harptown	28	37
Trumpetown	31	33
Violintown	37	43
TOTAL	215	217

Villages	Number of inhabitants
Clarinetown	1,508
Drumtown	56 more inhabitants than Violintown
Flutetown	386
Harptown	1456
Trumpetown	Three times more inhabitants than Flutetown
Violintown	Not provided

MOCK EXAM QUESTIONS

Q6.1 How many inhabitants are there in Violintown?

a. 1,254   **b.** 1,749   **c.** 2,157   **d.** 2,380   **e.** 2,856

Q6.2 By what percentage did the average expenditure per pupil across all villages increase between 2005 and 2006?

a. 0.93%   **b.** 1.75%   **c.** 2.70%   **d.** 3.13%   **e.** 4.06%

Q6.3 In 2005, the villages had opted to share the total costs for that year in proportion to the number of pupils in the school. By how much did Violintown's share of the costs increase between 2005 and 2006, to the nearest pound?

a. £273   **b.** £1,529   **c.** £2,046   **d.** £3,673   **e.** £4,965

Q6.4 In 2007, Trombonetown wants to join the school. It has a population of 1,724 and 23 of its children would be interested in becoming pupils. Assuming that the number of pupils from other villages does not vary, what proportion of the total population would be pupils of the school?

a. 1.74%   **b.** 1.83%   **c.** 1.96%   **d.** 2.00%   **e.** 2.05%

QR 7/10 Mock	It Rings a Bell

The Green Mobile Phone Company offers the following tariffs:

Tariff Number	Monthly Fee	Talk minutes included	SMS texts included
1	£15	0	Unlimited
2	£20	200	Unlimited
3	£35	600	Unlimited
4	£35	700	250
5	£45	900	Unlimited
6	£55	1500	Unlimited

Talk minutes included in the tariffs include calls to all mobile phones on the Green network but not calls to mobile phones on other networks. Texts included in the tariffs include texts sent to any mobile phone on any network. Calls and texts made outside of the tariff are charged as follows:

- Calls to Green mobile numbers: 15p per minute
- Calls to other mobiles: 40p per minute
- Additional text messages (any network): 10p per text

The H_2O Mobile Phone Company offers the following tariffs:

Tariff Number	Monthly Fee	Talk minutes Included	SMS texts included
A	£15	100	100
B	£20	200	200
C	£25	300	300
D	£30	700	400
E	£35	800	500
F	£40	1000	500

Talk minutes included in the tariffs include calls to mobiles on all networks (and not just H_2O). Texts can be sent to any mobile phone on any network. Calls and texts made outside of the tariff are charged as follows:

- Mobile numbers: 30p per minute
- Additional text messages: 12p per text

MOCK EXAM QUESTIONS

Q7.1 A Green Mobile Phone Company customer has opted for Tariff 4. In January, he had the following consumption:

- 300 talk minutes to contacts on the Green Telephone network
- 300 minutes to contacts who are on the H_2O network
- 100 texts to contacts on the Green Telephone network
- 150 texts to contacts who are on the H_2O network

How much was his telephone bill?

a. £35   **b.** £75   **c.** £125   **d.** £155   **e.** £183

Q7.2 A potential mobile customer is wondering which company and tariff he should be using. All his friends and family are using the Green Mobile Phone Company and he reckons he will be spending 10.5 hours on the phone to them every month and text them 450 times per month. Which tariff would ensure the cheapest bill?

a. Tariff 3   **b.** Tariff 4   **c.** Tariff C   **d.** Tariff D   **e.** Tariff E

Q7.3 A customer on Tariff E is thinking of moving to Tariff F. What is the minimum number of minutes that he would need to talk on the phone each month in order to make the move worthwhile?

a. 716 min   **b.** 717 min   **c.** 800 min   **d.** 816 min   **e.** 817 min

Q7.4 A customer on Tariff 6 has five friends to whom he has spoken as follows in one month (he spoke to no one else). His bill for the month is £450. The bill shows that he used the following minutes:

Jane	Green	220 minutes
John	H_2O	Illegible
Kelly	Green	280 minutes
Mark	Green	1000 minutes
Roberta	Green	500 minutes

How many minutes did he speak to John for that month?

a. 633   **b.** 800   **c.** 937   **d.** 1,275   **e.** 2,133

QR 8/10
Mock
Reward Scheme

A reward scheme works as follows:

- Clients can collect points from a range of retailers.
- Points are accumulated in a central account and can then be redeemed every quarter against a discount voucher. For every 250 points accumulated, the client receives a £2.50 voucher.
- Clients can decide to spend the vouchers in one of the retailers or can alternatively convert those vouchers into coach-miles vouchers which enable them to travel for free on any coach in the country up to the number of coach-miles they have accumulated.
- One voucher can be exchanged against 30 coach miles.

Retailers where points can be collected

Retailer	Points	Retailer	Points
The EC Electricity Company	1 point per £10 spent	**The GS Grocery Store**	1 point per £1 spent
The PS Petrol Station	4 points per £3 spent	**The FS Flower Shop**	1 point per £5 spent
The WS Wine Shop	1 points per £3 spent	**The SS Stationery shop**	3 points per £10 spent
The CR Car Rental company	1 point per £40 spent	**The JS Jewellery shop**	1 point per £35 spent

Notes

- Partial points cannot be granted. For example, a customer spending £47 on electricity will receive 4 points only and not 4.7 points.

- Only a multiple of 250 points can be converted into vouchers. For example, if a customer has accumulated 264 points, then 250 points will be converted into vouchers, whilst the remaining 14 will be carried forward to the next quarter.

MOCK EXAM QUESTIONS

Q8.1   In his first quarter with the scheme, a client spent the following:

- £45 Electricity
- £1,100 Grocery
- £423 Wine
- £50 Stationery

How many vouchers will he receive that quarter?

a. 4   **b.** 5   **c.** 6   **d.** 7   **e.** 8

Q8.2   A client wants to finance a 570-mile coach journey entirely with coach-miles obtained through the reward scheme. How much will he need to spend in electricity to acquire enough vouchers?

a. £47.50   **b.** £75   **c.** £475   **d.** 4,750   **e.** £47,500

Q8.3   What is the smallest amount that a client needs to spend in order to obtain vouchers worth £5?

a. £5   **b.** £375   **c.** £500   **d.** £775   **e.** £975

Q8.4   A customer obtained 30 coach-miles by spending £1250. Which type of products did he buy with that money?

a. Electricity **b.** Flowers   **c.** Jewellery **d.** Stationery **e.** Wine

QR 9/10
Mock
Topping It Up

Mrs Peacock is looking after several cats in the neighbourhood by leaving a large bowl of water outside her front door so that they can come to relieve their thirst whenever they want to.

The bowl has a capacity of 1.5 litres and every day at midnight she tops up the level of water so that the bowl is completely full. Some of the water that disappears from the bowl during the day is being drunk by the local cats; however, since the bowl is left outdoors, some of the water evaporates. The rate of evaporation differs depending on the season.

Daily evaporation rate depending on the month:

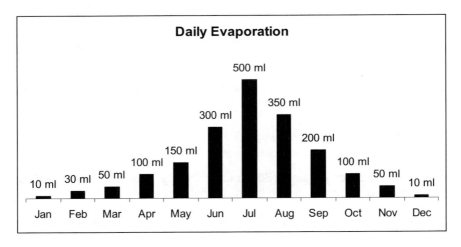

A cat drinks 75ml of water per day.
Assume there are 28 days in February.

MOCK EXAM QUESTIONS

Q9.1   On 10 August at 23:59, Mrs Peacock notices that the level of water left in the bowl is 1,000 ml. How many cats drank from the bowl in the past 24 hours?

a. 2   **b.** 3   **c.** 4   **d.** 5   **e.** 6

Q9.2   In February, 5 cats drank from the bowl every day. How much water in total did Mrs Peacock have to put in the bowl over the course of the month to replenish the level to the brim (in litres)?

a. 0.375   **b.** 0.840   **c.** 1.5   **d.** 11.34   **e.** 42

Q9.3   In July, Mrs Peacock noticed that, as well as the 12 cats who normally drink from the bowl in that month, some birds were also using the bowl's water to refresh themselves.

On 15 July at 23:59, there was no water left in the bowl. Assuming that the birds in question each drank 5ml of water from the bowl, how many birds drank from the bowl on that day?

a. 0 birds   **b.** 12 birds   **c.** 20 birds   **d.** 100 birds   **e.** 120 birds

Q9.4   What is the average daily evaporation rate for the last three months of the year (expressed in ml/day)?

a. 30   **b.** 50   **c.** 50.28   **d.** 53.33   **e.** 53.37

305

QR 10/10 Mock	League Table

A local authority published the following table of 'A' Level results for the entire region. The table shows the percentage of A grades obtained, as well as the percentage of grades A & B combined, measured in relation to the total number of 'A' Levels taken.

School	Number of candidates	Number of A Levels taken	% A	% A + B combined
Springwood	154	450	80%	94%
Rosamund	74	270	30%	70%
Tootham	95	380	80%	90%
Woodworm	137	280	80%	85%
Harringstone	105	320	50%	60%
TOTAL	**565**	**1700**		

MOCK EXAM QUESTIONS

Q10.1 How many 'A' Levels taken by Rosamund students were obtained at Grade B?

    a. 30   **b.** 40   **c.** 74   **d.** 108   **e.** 270

Q10.2 When considering all A Levels taken across all five schools together, what is the percentage of 'A' Levels for which non-A grades were obtained?

    a. 4.59%   **b.** 6.09%   **c.** 9.79%   **d.** 18.59%   **e.** 33.59%

Q10.3 All Tootham students took the same number of 'A' Levels. The school has a boy:girl ratio of 40:60. How many 'A' Levels did the girls take in total?

    a. 57   **b.** 152   **c.** 178   **d.** 228   **e.** 300

Q10.4 At Harringstone, 30 students only took 1 'A' Level. How many 'A' Levels did the rest of the students take on average?

    a. 2.76   **b.** 3.05   **c.** 3.87   **d.** 4.01   **e.** 4.23

MOCK EXAM

ABSTRACT REASONING

(13 sets of 5 test shapes – 15 minutes)

AR 1/13
Mock
Test Shapes 1.1 to 1.5

Set A **Set B**

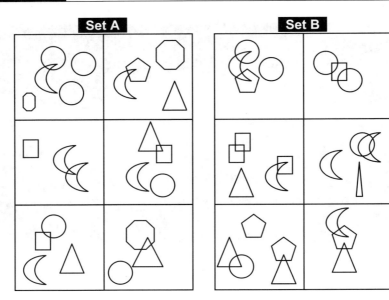

To which of the two sets above do the following shapes belong?

Shape 1.1 **Shape 1.2** **Shape 1.3** **Shape 1.4** **Shape 1.5**

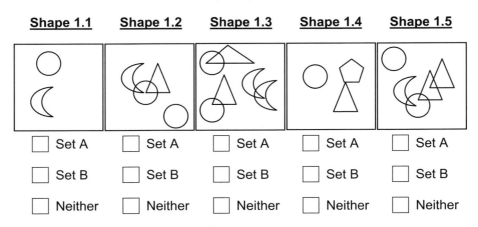

☐ Set A	☐ Set A	☐ Set A	☐ Set A	☐ Set A
☐ Set B	☐ Set B	☐ Set B	☐ Set B	☐ Set B
☐ Neither	☐ Neither	☐ Neither	☐ Neither	☐ Neither

AR 2/13 Mock — Test Shapes 2.1 to 2.5

Set A

Set B

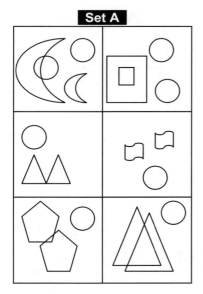
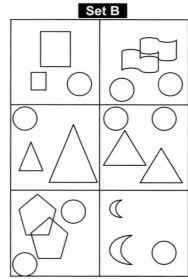

To which of the two sets above do the following shapes belong?

Shape 2.1	Shape 2.2	Shape 2.3	Shape 2.4	Shape 2.5

☐ Set A ☐ Set A ☐ Set A ☐ Set A ☐ Set A

☐ Set B ☐ Set B ☐ Set B ☐ Set B ☐ Set B

☐ Neither ☐ Neither ☐ Neither ☐ Neither ☐ Neither

AR 3/13
Mock
Test Shapes 3.1 to 3.5

Set A

Set B

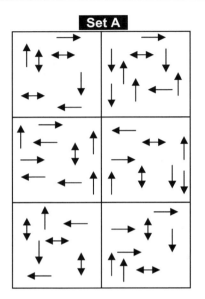
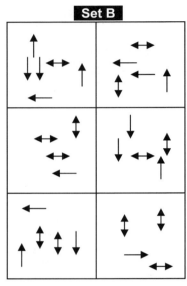

To which of the two sets above do the following shapes belong?

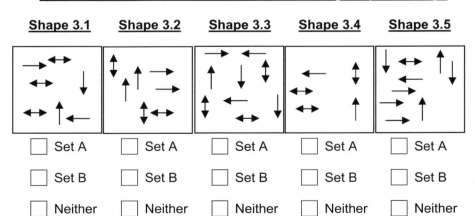

Shape 3.1	Shape 3.2	Shape 3.3	Shape 3.4	Shape 3.5
☐ Set A	☐ Set A	☐ Set A	☐ Set A	☐ Set A
☐ Set B	☐ Set B	☐ Set B	☐ Set B	☐ Set B
☐ Neither	☐ Neither	☐ Neither	☐ Neither	☐ Neither

AR 4/13 Mock	Test Shapes 4.1 to 4.5

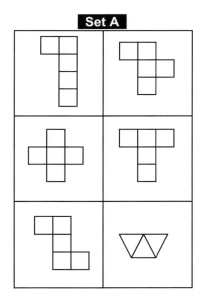

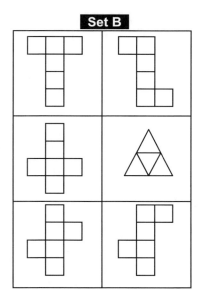

To which of the two sets above do the following shapes belong?

Shape 4.1	Shape 4.2	Shape 4.3	Shape 4.4	Shape 4.5

☐ Set A	☐ Set A	☐ Set A	☐ Set A	☐ Set A
☐ Set B	☐ Set B	☐ Set B	☐ Set B	☐ Set B
☐ Neither	☐ Neither	☐ Neither	☐ Neither	☐ Neither

AR 5/13
Mock
Test Shapes 5.1 to 5.5

Set A

Set B

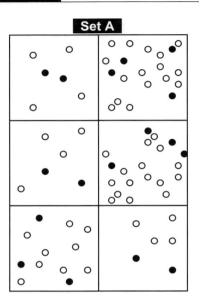
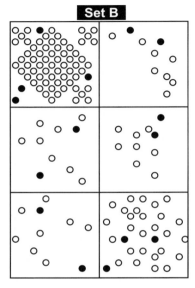

To which of the two sets above do the following shapes belong?

Shape 5.1	Shape 5.2	Shape 5.3	Shape 5.4	Shape 5.5

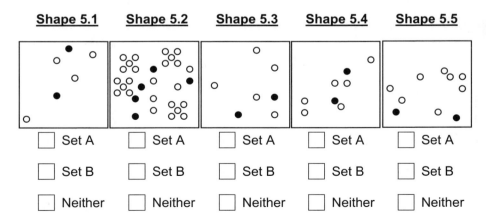

	Set A		Set A		Set A		Set A		Set A
	Set B		Set B		Set B		Set B		Set B
	Neither		Neither		Neither		Neither		Neither

AR 6/13 Mock	Test Shapes 6.1 to 6.5

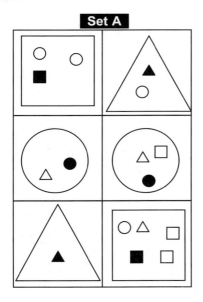

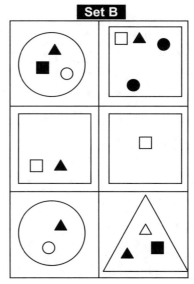

To which of the two sets above do the following shapes belong?

Shape 6.1	Shape 6.2	Shape 6.3	Shape 6.4	Shape 6.5

☐ Set A   ☐ Set A   ☐ Set A   ☐ Set A   ☐ Set A

☐ Set B   ☐ Set B   ☐ Set B   ☐ Set B   ☐ Set B

☐ Neither   ☐ Neither   ☐ Neither   ☐ Neither   ☐ Neither

AR 7/13 Mock — Test Shapes 7.1 to 7.5

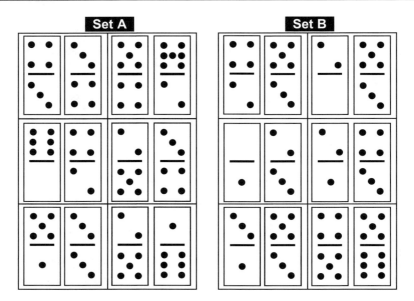

Set A   **Set B**

To which of the two sets above do the following shapes belong?

Shape 7.1   **Shape 7.2**   **Shape 7.3**   **Shape 7.4**   **Shape 7.5**

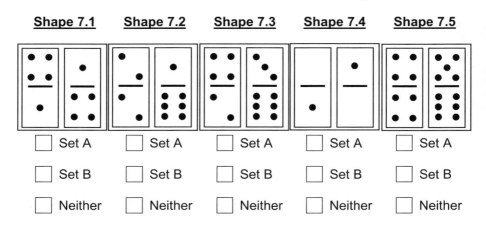

Shape 7.1	Shape 7.2	Shape 7.3	Shape 7.4	Shape 7.5
☐ Set A	☐ Set A	☐ Set A	☐ Set A	☐ Set A
☐ Set B	☐ Set B	☐ Set B	☐ Set B	☐ Set B
☐ Neither	☐ Neither	☐ Neither	☐ Neither	☐ Neither

AR 8/13 Mock	Test Shapes 8.1 to 8.5

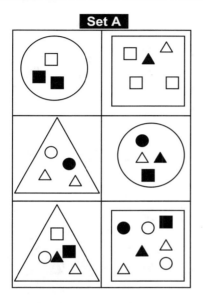

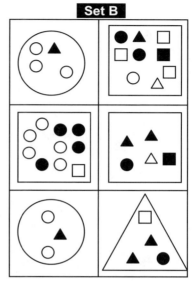

To which of the two sets above do the following shapes belong?

Shape 8.1   Shape 8.2   Shape 8.3   Shape 8.4   Shape 8.5

☐ Set A   ☐ Set A   ☐ Set A   ☐ Set A   ☐ Set A

☐ Set B   ☐ Set B   ☐ Set B   ☐ Set B   ☐ Set B

☐ Neither   ☐ Neither   ☐ Neither   ☐ Neither   ☐ Neither

AR 9/13
Mock
Test Shapes 9.1 to 9.5

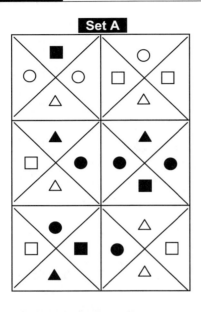
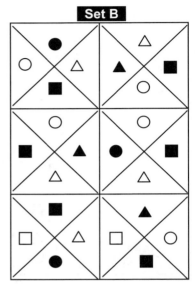

Set A

Set B

To which of the two sets above do the following shapes belong?

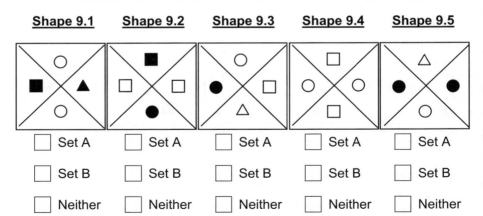

Shape 9.1   Shape 9.2   Shape 9.3   Shape 9.4   Shape 9.5

☐ Set A   ☐ Set A   ☐ Set A   ☐ Set A   ☐ Set A

☐ Set B   ☐ Set B   ☐ Set B   ☐ Set B   ☐ Set B

☐ Neither   ☐ Neither   ☐ Neither   ☐ Neither   ☐ Neither

AR 10/13 Mock — Test Shapes 10.1 to 10.5

Set A

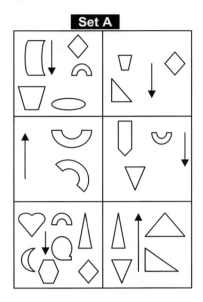

Set B

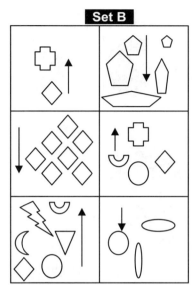

To which of the two sets above do the following shapes belong?

Shape 10.1	Shape 10.2	Shape10.3	Shape 10.4	Shape 10.5

☐ Set A   ☐ Set A   ☐ Set A   ☐ Set A   ☐ Set A

☐ Set B   ☐ Set B   ☐ Set B   ☐ Set B   ☐ Set B

☐ Neither   ☐ Neither   ☐ Neither   ☐ Neither   ☐ Neither

AR 11/13
Mock
Test Shapes 11.1 to 11.5

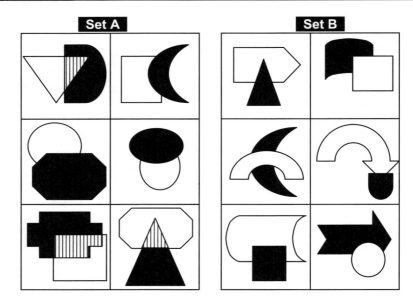

To which of the two sets above do the following shapes belong?

Shape 11.1	Shape 11.2	Shape 11.3	Shape 11.4	Shape 11.5

☐ Set A   ☐ Set A   ☐ Set A   ☐ Set A   ☐ Set A

☐ Set B   ☐ Set B   ☐ Set B   ☐ Set B   ☐ Set B

☐ Neither   ☐ Neither   ☐ Neither   ☐ Neither   ☐ Neither

Test Shapes 12.1 to 12.5

Set A	Set B

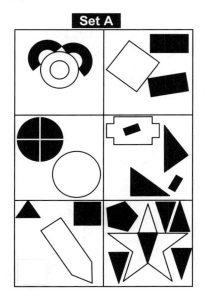 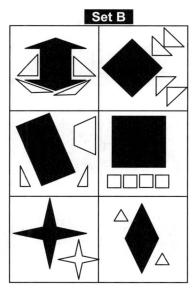

To which of the two sets above do the following shapes belong?

Shape 12.1 **Shape 12.2** **Shape 12.3** **Shape 12.4** **Shape 12.5**

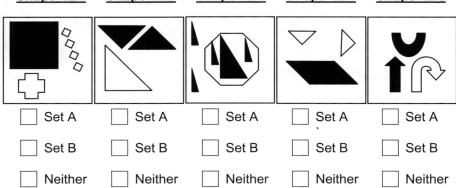

Set A	Set A	Set A	Set A	Set A
Set B	Set B	Set B	Set B	Set B
Neither	Neither	Neither	Neither	Neither

AR 13/13
Mock
Test Shapes 13.1 to 13.5

Set A **Set B**

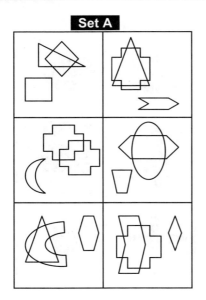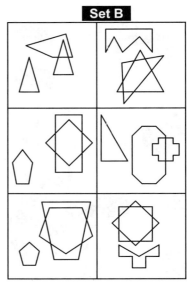

To which of the two sets above do the following shapes belong?

Shape 13.1　　**Shape 13.2**　　**Shape 13.3**　　**Shape 13.4**　　**Shape 13.5**

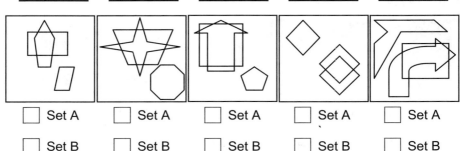

☐ Set A　　☐ Set A　　☐ Set A　　☐ Set A　　☐ Set A

☐ Set B　　☐ Set B　　☐ Set B　　☐ Set B　　☐ Set B

☐ Neither　☐ Neither　☐ Neither　☐ Neither　☐ Neither

MOCK EXAM
VERBAL REASONING
(11 sets of 4 questions – 21 minutes)

VR 1/11 Mock	Christmas Repeats

TEXT

Television viewers have grown increasingly discontent about the number of repeats in TV schedules during the Christmas period. However, despite sometimes very vocal negative publicity both from members of the public and from politicians, broadcasters have done little to modify their programme grids. The number of repeats over Christmas 2007, taking into account all channels, was 25% higher than over Christmas 2006. In a survey, Channel 5 came out worst with 60% of programmes in its grid being repeats, whilst BBC1 came out best with only 16% of its programmes being repeats. Channel 4 was the only terrestrial broadcaster that had not increased the percentage of repeats in relation to the overall number of programmes shown.

Representatives of the Liberal Democrats political party argued that an abuse of repeats would make people switch off their TV sets at Christmas. Members of family groups suggested that switching off the TV would have a positive impact on family life by encouraging children and parents to spend more time together. Broadcasters responded with their own survey, demonstrating that actually members of the public enjoyed watching old films and repeats of their favourite programmes, in part because it made them relive their own childhood and they could share their memories with their children.

In 2007, viewing share for BBC1 fell from 25.5% in 2006 to 22% in 2007, BBC2's share fell from 11.9% to 8.5%, ITV1's share fell from 20.8% to 19.3%, Channel 4's share fell by more than 11% to 8.7%, whilst Channel 5's share fell from 8.8% to 5.5%.

MOCK EXAM QUESTIONS

Q1.1 In 2007, the number of repeats on Channel 5 was higher than the number of repeats on BBC1.

☐ True

☐ False

☐ Can't tell

Q1.2 The number of repeats on Channel 4 in 2007 was the same as in 2006.

☐ True

☐ False

☐ Can't tell

Q1.3 Decreasing the proportion of repeats would make viewers go back to terrestrial channels.

☐ True

☐ False

☐ Can't tell

Q1.4 In 2006, Channel 4 was more popular than BBC2.

☐ True

☐ False

☐ Can't tell

VR 2/11
Mock
HIV Vaccine

TEXT

In a recent media interview, Professor Luc Montagnier, the French virologist who, with his team, first identified the HIV virus in 1983 and obtained the Nobel Prize in 2008, explained that he hoped to develop a therapeutic vaccine for HIV within the next four years. Whilst efforts to develop a preventative vaccine (i.e. a vaccine administered to healthy people to stop them getting infected in the first place) have proved unsuccessful so far, a therapeutic vaccine (i.e. a vaccine administered to already-infected patients designed to help them fight the consequences of the infection and therefore reduce suffering) looks far more promising.

Luc Montagnier explains: "Currently, there are many treatments available for HIV once it has been diagnosed, but they are burdensome and toxic because they have to be taken every day. As a result, intolerances can develop in the long term and some patients may develop resistance to the virus. These treatments can also be very expensive. Therefore the aim, eventually, is to be able to do without the treatments. This could be achieved by encouraging the immune system to fight the virus. We know this is possible because there already are people who are naturally resisting against the effects of the infection and the illness, i.e. who are infected but not ill. If a therapeutic vaccine is developed, the patient will first need to start with the combination therapy to reduce the virus load. Thereafter, the risk will need to be taken to stop the therapy and to start the vaccination. If the vaccine fails, the patient will always have the option to revert to the combination therapy."

The French scientist also stated that, although some people may not have the HIV virus in their blood, they see their immune system continue to fail. "These people are still infected. However, although the virus may have disappeared from the blood, it remains hidden in organs and tissues, where it can restart as soon as treatment has been stopped. That is what we call the reservoir of the virus. The aim of our research is to analyse that reservoir and to find a treatment that will totally eliminate the virus or at least make it less harmful for the patient."

MOCK EXAM QUESTIONS

Q2.1 The new vaccine currently being researched by Professor Montagnier should prevent currently non-HIV-infected patients from becoming infected if they ever come into contact with the HIV virus.

☐ True

☐ False

☐ Can't tell

Q2.2 The reservoir is a barrier to the eradication of a virus.

☐ True

☐ False

☐ Can't tell

Q2.3 Patients who are administered the therapeutic vaccine will no longer need combination therapy.

☐ True

☐ False

☐ Can't tell

Q2.4 It is impossible to develop a preventative vaccine for HIV.

☐ True

☐ False

☐ Can't tell

VR 3/11 Mock	E–Cigarettes

TEXT

Electronic cigarettes are being sold on the internet and in a number of high-street shops to smokers wishing to avoid the dangers of smoking. Some of these "e-cigarettes" contain toxic substances. Some also contain nicotine but are not officially recognised as substitutes for the more traditional smoking-cessation methods. Since the results of a thorough investigation are still being awaited, the health authorities are encouraging potential users to remain prudent.

E-cigarettes look like real cigarettes, taste of tobacco and even give out smoke – this makes it very appealing to smokers. Additional asset: it can be used in public places such as restaurants. But what is it exactly? In reality, the e-cigarette does not produce any real smoke but a vapour charged with aromatic essences. The device is made up of a metal tube containing an electronic circuit, a battery and a cartridge containing a liquid. When the user draws his first puff, the microprocessor activates a device which mixes the air inhaled by the user with a warm vapour. Problem: the liquid held in the cartridge contains chemicals that can be harmful such as glycol propylene (which can cause neurological effects similar to drunkenness), linalol and menthol (both of which can cause convulsions, particular in the elderly and those with epilepsy).

Beyond the toxicity of the e-cigarette, the health authorities oppose other issues with the manufacturers, specifically the fact that e-cigarettes containing nicotine are being advertised as smoking-cessation devices: a claim which is illegal under current regulations as no licence was obtained to commercialise the product. Such a licence is compulsory for all nicotine substitutes, but can be lengthy and costly to obtain. "We do not have the size or the means to make such a request," says a representative of the main manufacturer. "We await the results of the studies being currently undertaken to determine whether we can continue to commercialise this product."

MOCK EXAM QUESTIONS

Q3.1 If approved, e-cigarettes will remove the dangers of passive smoking.

☐ True

☐ False

☐ Can't tell

Q3.2 The e-cigarette is safe for a young person who is not epileptic.

☐ True

☐ False

☐ Can't tell

Q3.3 In the future, e-cigarettes could be used to encourage smokers to give up smoking.

☐ True

☐ False

☐ Can't tell

Q3.4 E-cigarettes are currently illegal.

☐ True

☐ False

☐ Can't tell

VR 4/11 Mock	NICE

TEXT

The National Institute for Health and Clinical Excellence (NICE) has recently announced that it would increase the threshold at which drugs are deemed to be too expensive to be made available to patients. NICE's role is to decide which drugs can be prescribed to patients under the NHS based on efficacy and cost. Until recently, NICE, whose decisions are binding, would not approve any drug with an annual cost of more than £30,000 per patient. The proposed increase in this threshold will only apply in certain cases, for example when a patient has a life expectancy of 2 years or less and where it can be demonstrated that the treatment will extend life by a significant amount of time (usually taken as 3 months). This may benefit many cancer patients.

In the past, NICE has been the subject of several controversies and criticisms. The main reproach is that NICE puts a price on life and is being seen as a rationing body. NICE is a body which reviews evidence in the context of value for money. It therefore has to balance efficacy and cost. This means that some treatments which could add a lot of value to a patient are discounted because they are too expensive. Rationing is important because the budget is finite and because there are newer and more expensive treatments every day. However, patients can feel that they are being denied the best treatment. It is a dilemma which is difficult to resolve in a cost-controlled environment. It should be remembered that NICE only deals with the provision of treatment or care in the NHS. NICE decisions do not apply in the private sector and patients can access non-approved treatments if they pay for them privately. NICE has also been criticised for being slow to reach decisions (up to 2 years). Whilst a treatment or procedure is in the process of being reviewed, it is left to the initiative of each Trust to decide whether it wishes to fund the treatment being reviewed. Different Trusts make different decisions, which leads to inequalities of care. In a recent report, Lord Darzi, Health Minister, has recommended that the approval time should be reduced to 3 months, which should improve access to care.

MOCK EXAM QUESTIONS

Q4.1 In future, NICE will be required to make decisions in 3 months instead of up to 2 years.

☐ True

☐ False

☐ Can't tell

Q4.2 Currently, patients cannot receive treatment in the UK unless that treatment costs under £30,000.

☐ True

☐ False

☐ Can't tell

Q4.3 Some NHS patients are denied the most effective treatment available simply on the basis of cost.

☐ True

☐ False

☐ Can't tell

Q4.4 NICE decisions lead to inequalities of care within the NHS.

☐ True

☐ False

☐ Can't tell

VR 5/11 Mock exam	Heavy Metal

TEXT

A recent English study published in the *Chemistry Central Journal* reveals that most of the wines sold around the world contain excessive doses of heavy metals. Declan Naughton and Andrea Petroczi, from Kingston University have analysed wines produced in sixteen countries, demonstrating that only Argentinean, Brazilian and Italian wines have low concentrations of heavy metals. French wines are not well ranked, followed in decreasing order by Austria, Spain, Germany, and Portugal. Hungarian and Slovakian wines contain the highest levels. In order to reach these conclusions, the English researchers analysed a wide range of scientific studies showing the quantities of metal present in wines. To the data they then applied a new risk evaluation index linked to the long-term exposure to chemical pollutants; this index, named Target Hazard Quotient (THQ), was originally designed in the US by the Environmental Protection Agency. Their calculations, based on an average daily consumption of a quarter of a litre of wine over a period of time from the age of 18 to the age of 82, show that the THQ index was between 50 and 200 for the majority of wines, and going up to 300 for Hungarian and Slovakian wines. The most worrying doses relate to metals such as manganese, copper and vanadium.

Reactions to this study are very diverse. Some scientists believe that, even though the study highlights a potential risk only, it does encourage the scientific community to ask questions about the role and potential effect on health of elements which are rarely considered by studies. Others state that the presence of minerals in wine does not mean that these are being assimilated into the body. Some American studies have also shown that there exists a substance in wine – named rhamnogalacturonan – which envelops and neutralises metallic elements.

MOCK EXAM QUESTIONS

Q5.1 The THQ index is a measure of the concentration level of heavy metals.

☐ True

☐ False

☐ Can't tell

Q5.2 The concentration of heavy metals is higher in Portuguese wines than in Spanish wines.

☐ True

☐ False

☐ Can't tell

Q5.3 Wines with high concentrations of heavy metals are dangerous for human health.

☐ True

☐ False

☐ Can't tell

Q5.4 The scientists who published the study have reached their conclusions by questioning wine drinkers in sixteen countries.

☐ True

☐ False

☐ Can't tell

VR 6/11 Mock — Women in Ancient Egypt

TEXT

The fact that Cleopatra held such a prominent position as Pharaoh is indicative of the fact that women played a prominent role in the building of Ancient Egypt from the early times. Unlike in most other ancient civilizations (including Rome and Greece), there is strong evidence that Egyptian women enjoyed the same legal and economic rights as the Egyptian man. This notion is reflected in Egyptian art and historical inscriptions. Such gender equality stems from the fact that Egyptian national identity would have derived from all people sharing a common relationship with the king. In this relationship, which all men and women shared equally, they were in a sense equal to each other. This is not to say that Egypt was an egalitarian society. Legal distinctions in Egypt were based much more upon differences in the social classes, rather than differences in gender. Rights and privileges were not uniform from one class to another but, within the given classes, it seems that equal economic and legal rights were, for the most part, accorded to both men and women.

We know that women could manage and dispose of private property (including land, slaves, servants and money); they could also inherit one-third of community property (i.e. property accrued by them and their husband during the marriage) on the death of their husband, with the remaining two-thirds being distributed amongst the children. They had the right to take others to court, and, more importantly, we know that there was no discrimination against women in the allocation of jobs; for example, there were over a hundred female doctors in Ancient Egypt. Women could and did hold male administrative positions in Egypt. However, such cases are few, and thus appear to be the exceptions to tradition. Given the relative scarcity of such cases, they might reflect extraordinary individuals in unusual circumstances. The Egyptian woman in general was free to go about in public; she worked out in the fields and in estate workshops. Certainly, she did not wear a veil, which is first documented among the ancient Assyrians (perhaps reflecting a tradition of the ancient Semitic-speaking people of the Syrian and Arabian deserts). However, it was perhaps unsafe for an Egyptian woman to venture far from her town alone.

MOCK EXAM QUESTIONS

Q6.1 It was unsafe for Egyptian women to travel away from their home town.

☐ True

☐ False

☐ Can't tell

Q6.2 In a family comprising a man, his wife and two children, on the death of the husband, each child would get one-third of the property.

☐ True

☐ False

☐ Can't tell

Q6.3 There were more female doctors than female administrators in Ancient Egypt.

☐ True

☐ False

☐ Can't tell

Q6.4 Egypt was a fair and classless society.

☐ True

☐ False

☐ Can't tell

VR 7/11
Mock
The Eye of the World

TEXT

In the past 18 years, the famous Americano-European spatial telescope in service since 24 April 1990 has revolutionised our knowledge of space. As is often the case in great epics, its beginnings were chaotic. The catastrophe of the shuttle Challenger in 1986 delayed the launch for several years. Then, once in orbit, scientists discovered with much consternation that their best instrument, which cost the meagre amount of 2 billion dollars was … short-sighted. The blame is firmly placed on a small defect on the main mirror, which a team of astronauts on board the shuttle Endeavour would correct 3 years later. Since then, thanks to three further maintenance NASA missions, Hubble has had an almost faultless career, collecting no fewer than 800,000 exclusive images of space, some of which are of a rare beauty and have gone round the world.

Still, as astronomer Julianne Dalcanton of the University of Washington remarks in a recent article published in the journal *Nature*, "Many people would be surprised to learn that Hubble's size is relatively modest in comparison to some of the more modern telescopes." Indeed, the diameter of its mirror (2.4 metres) is four times smaller than those of the four telescopes located in the Atacama Desert in northern Chile. Furthermore, some of its instruments are over a decade old. Despite this, Hubble has gathered images which are ten times more precise than those obtained with ground-based telescopes. Hubble's success is due to the fact that it orbits nearly 350 miles above the Earth, far removed from the atmosphere and ambient light that limits the effectiveness of ground-based telescopes, and the upcoming servicing mission will likely allow Hubble to add to its already rich legacy of scientific discovery. Indeed, the renowned telescope is preparing for its final chapter, starting with the launch of the space shuttle Atlantis on 12 May 2009 for NASA's fifth and final service mission to the telescope.

MOCK EXAM QUESTIONS

Q7.1 Hubble is the fifth biggest earth-bound telescope.

☐ True

☐ False

☐ Can't tell

Q7.2 Telescopes with smaller sized mirrors provide better quality pictures.

☐ True

☐ False

☐ Can't tell

Q7.3 The images produced by Hubble before the initial repairs were of better quality than those currently produced by the telescopes in the Chilean desert.

☐ True

☐ False

☐ Can't tell

Q7.4 Some of Hubble's instruments were replaced or added during some of the service missions.

☐ True

☐ False

☐ Can't tell

VR 8/11 Mock	Green Fly

TEXT

An Air New Zealand (ANZ) Boeing 747 was the first plane to fly last week using a mix of kerosene and of a biofuel of so-called "second generation", during which one of its four engines flew on fuel containing 50% of a diester made from jatropha oil. All airlines are aware of the limits of first generation biofuels (made from sugar cane, soya, rapeseed or corn): some have freezing temperatures which are too high; their culture is accused of interfering with fertile soils which should be reserved for food destined for human consumption; and they encourage deforestation. Consequently, ANZ is keen to reassure that it will respect three non-negotiable criteria: the culture of any biofuel used should not interfere with food cultures; the use of the fuel should not lead to any technical modifications of the planes; and it should remain competitive with kerosene and be available immediately.

The jatropha oil was collected in India, Malawi, Mozambique and Tanzania, where it is already used to make soap and lamp oil for local markets. The plant, native to South America, can be grown on very dry soil and is not edible, meaning that its culture should not compete with food cultures. Jatropha sounds a promising opportunity: its seeds can contain up to 40% of oil and it has been said that one hectare could produce 2 tons of the plant – enough to power a Boeing 747 for over 100km. However, the first trials to extract the oil have been disappointing and some growers – particularly in Ghana – have shown reticence to start growing the plant given the high level of manpower required and the uncertainty surrounding its use, which would make them financially dependent on the fuel refineries. In addition, some researchers have expressed concerns about the toxicity of the plant, which could have an impact on human health.

Jatropha is not the only biofuel studied by the airline industry. In February 2008, Boeing and Virgin Atlantic did a trial flight with a mix of palm oil and coconut oil only. Environmentalists criticised the flight as a publicity stunt, arguing that these oils cannot be produced in sufficient quantities in the long term to support all airlines.

MOCK EXAM QUESTIONS

Q8.1 No plane can fly using 100% biofuel.

☐ True

☐ False

☐ Can't tell

Q8.2 Jatropha cannot grow on soil normally used for growing food.

☐ True

☐ False

☐ Can't tell

Q8.3 Using jatropha would not lead to deforestation.

☐ True

☐ False

☐ Can't tell

Q8.4 Biofuel is greener than conventional fuel.

☐ True

☐ False

☐ Can't tell

VR 9/11 Mock	Unwanted Goods

TEXT

Dear Mrs Ackroyd,

Many thanks for your complaint email about our online teapot shop. I would like to use this opportunity to emphasise that we are one of the leading providers of teapots in the country and as such we always seek to ensure that our customers are fully satisfied with the services that we offer.

I see from our records that you ordered a special teapot suitable for use in a dishwasher on 2 April, which you say you received on 4 April, and I understand from your email that you now wish to cancel the order as someone else has already bought this item on your behalf. The purchase of goods from online shops such as ours is regulated by the Distance Selling Regulations 2000 which state that:

- You can cancel your order within 7 full days following receipt of the item. The retailer must accept your cancellation whatever your reasons and provide a full refund. Should the item be returned in a damaged state, the retailer is entitled to make a deduction proportionate to the loss incurred as a result. Online retailers may also make a deduction for any credit card and administration fees incurred, though this is not our policy.

- Retailers have no obligation to accept an order cancellation past this 7-day period though, in our case, we have decided to extend this right to our customers for a full period of 14 days. Our policy is that, after this extended period, we do not grant customers any refunds, whatever the reason for their request.

I would like to thank you personally for returning the teapot undamaged; however, in view of the above, we cannot accept the cancellation of your order and are therefore unable to grant you any refund whatsoever.

Best regards
Ron Donaldson, Customer Service Manager

MOCK EXAM QUESTIONS

Q9.1 One of the reasons for not granting Mrs Ackroyd's refund was that her excuse to cancel the order is not valid.

☐ True

☐ False

☐ Can't tell

Q9.2 Mrs Ackroyd's complaint email was sent on or after 19 April.

☐ True

☐ False

☐ Can't tell

Q9.3 Under the Distance Selling Regulations, it is never possible to receive a full refund.

☐ True

☐ False

☐ Can't tell

Q9.4 Generally speaking, if a customer orders an item from an online retailer on 1 July then, assuming that the online retailer has no special policy providing better terms than the Distance Selling Regulations 2004, the online retailer has no obligation to grant any refund if the order is cancelled after 8 July.

☐ True

☐ False

☐ Can't tell

VR 10/11
Mock
The Veggie Diet

TEXT

Contrary to common wisdom, being a vegetarian is not unhealthy. Scientists have now identified that the exclusion of animal flesh from our diet (both from meat or fish) does not lead to deficiencies, provided the right cereals are added to the diet, as these will provide most of the required protein intake.

With regard to Vitamin B12, exclusively present in foods of animal origin, eating dairy products or milk can help the vegetarian avoid any deficiency. However, vegans (i.e. vegetarians who eat neither dairy products nor eggs) risk developing a Vitamin B12 deficiency and therefore anaemia. And we are not even talking about the calcium that such foods bring into the diet! Vegans must therefore opt for vegetables and fruits rich in calcium such as cress, spinach, almond, hazelnuts or pistachio nuts.

Several epidemiological studies have demonstrated that vegetarians are less prone to hypertension and coronary comorbidity, not only because of the quantity and nature of the lipids they ingest, i.e. less saturated fats, but also lifestyle habits (little alcohol or tobacco and greater physical activity), which are responsible for these health benefits. In addition, fibres create short-chain fatty acids which slow down cholesterol synthesis.

Vegetarians also win on the issues of obesity; research shows that the proportion of vegetarians who are obese is less than the proportion of non-vegetarians who are obese. The prominence of fibre in vegetarian diets makes people feel full more quickly and vegetarians therefore tend to eat smaller quantities. A reduction of the incidence of some cancers in vegetarians can primarily be explained by a significant consumption of fruits and vegetables. Not counting that the presence of numerous anti-oxidants in plants is supposed to have anti-carcinogenic virtues, although this has never been proven.

MOCK EXAM QUESTIONS

Q10.1   A patient with anaemia will also have Vitamin B12 deficiency.

☐ True

☐ False

☐ Can't tell

Q10.2   Cress is a good source of calcium and Vitamin B12 for vegans.

☐ True

☐ False

☐ Can't tell

Q10.3   Vegetarians are less prone to lung cancer than non-vegetarians.

☐ True

☐ False

☐ Can't tell

Q10.4   Most obese people are non-vegetarians.

☐ True

☐ False

☐ Can't tell

VR 11/11
Mock

Pole Position

TEXT

Should we be worried if we have a mobile phone mast (or pole) above our head? Without bearing any judgement on the negative effects of radio frequencies, a new study by the French National Centre for Scientific Research (CNRS) shows that the exposure to waves is stronger at a distance than underneath or near the pole.

In the course of the study, 200 people carried personal radiation badges which recorded the exposure to radio frequencies for 24 hours at different distances from the mobile phone pole depending on personal movements during the day.

Firstly, the study showed that the exposure to radio frequencies was at its maximum at a distance of approximately 280 metres from the pole, especially in urban areas. In the areas immediately adjoining urban areas, the maximum exposure to radio frequencies was at a distance of 1 kilometre. The study also shows that the exposure varied considerably even at identical distances from the pole.

Secondly, the electric field measured remained constant below 1.5 V/m, therefore below international norms. However, those norms are judged insufficient by a number of militant groups who lobby for a reduction to 0.6 V/m.

The French Academy of Medicine published a report in March stating that it knows no mechanism by which electromagnetic fields in this range of energy and frequency could have a negative effect on health.

MOCK EXAM QUESTIONS

Q11.1 Both the report issued by the CNRS and the French Academy of Medicine state that radiofrequencies have no effect on health.

☐ True

☐ False

☐ Can't tell

Q11.2 The level of radiation received by an individual is proportionate to the distance from the pole.

☐ True

☐ False

☐ Can't tell

Q11.3 People living near mobile phone masts in rural areas are less exposed than those living in urban areas.

☐ True

☐ False

☐ Can't tell

Q11.4 The international norm for electric field exposure is above 0.6 V/m.

☐ True

☐ False

☐ Can't tell

MOCK EXAM

DECISION ANALYSIS

(1 code with 26 questions – 29 minutes)

CODE		
A = Personal	1 = Sound	✪ = Smooth
B = Opposite	2 = Food	✤ = Wet
C = Increase	3 = Textile	ψ = Empty
D = Extreme	4 = Size	♣ = Closed
E = Plural	5 = Furniture	♦ = Safe
F = Circumstance	6 = Ground	♥ = Green
G = Future	7 = Wealth	● = Big
J = Accept	8 = Man	∇ = Special
K = Introduce	9 = Sleep	
L = Again	10 = Room	
M = Use	11 = Glass	
N = Regular	12 = Light	
	13 = Quality	
	14 = Container	
	15 = Heat	
	16 = Wish	

What is the best interpretation of the following coded messages?

Q1:   (3, 5, 9), D4

- [ ] **A.** The duvet is too big
- [ ] **B.** My bed takes up too much space
- [ ] **C.** Your sleeping bag is too big for me
- [ ] **D.** The bed sheet is too large for me
- [ ] **E.** My tailor is rich

Q2:   BA, (✤10, 3), ✤

- [ ] **A.** My shower curtain is dry
- [ ] **B.** Your soap is wet
- [ ] **C.** Your towel is not dry
- [ ] **D.** The bathroom floor needs mopping up
- [ ] **E.** Your face cloth needs to dry

Q3:   (11, ❖10), B⊗

- A. The shower screen is missing
- B. The bath taps are dirty
- C. The bathroom window is frosted
- D. The shaving mirror is old
- E. Your bathroom light is flickering

Q4:   (A, 9, 10, 3), DBC, 12

- A. My bedroom carpet is getting dirty
- B. My blanket is too thin
- C. The bedroom rug is wearing out
- D. The bedroom curtains are very pale
- E. My bedroom curtains block out the sun

Q5:   (8, 11⊗), C7, F❖

- A. The plumber wears expensive glasses
- B. Cleaning windows costs more after heavy rain
- C. The glazier charges more in the winter
- D. The window cleaner gets paid more when it rains
- E. Men who wear glasses clean them more often when it rains

Q6:   A, (C, 13, 9), (F, 12)

- A. I sleep little but well
- B. I sleep better with the light on
- C. It is better to sleep with the light on
- D. I sleep more in the summer
- E. In the summer I have a good siesta

CODE		
A = Personal	1 = Sound	✿ = Smooth
B = Opposite	2 = Food	❖ = Wet
C = Increase	3 = Textile	ψ = Empty
D = Extreme	4 = Size	♣ = Closed
E = Plural	5 = Furniture	♦ = Safe
F = Circumstance	6 = Ground	♥ = Green
G = Future	7 = Wealth	● = Big
J = Accept	8 = Man	∇ = Special
K = Introduce	9 = Sleep	
L = Again	10 = Room	
M = Use	11 = Glass	
N = Regular	12 = Light	
	13 = Quality	
	14 = Container	
	15 = Heat	
	16 = Wish	

Q7:   **8, BA10, D1, AB9**

- ☐ **A.** My neighbour's constant noise keeps me awake
- ☐ **B.** My husband's snoring stops me from sleeping
- ☐ **C.** Men find it difficult to sleep in my bedroom
- ☐ **D.** Sleeping can be hard when you have neighbours who party all the time
- ☐ **E.** I don't sleep well when my neighbour is too noisy

Q8:   **(2, 10, ❖5), Bψ, E(11, 14)**

- ☐ **A.** The glasses cabinet has watermarks
- ☐ **B.** The kitchen tap is clogged up with limescale
- ☐ **C.** I spilt water on the kitchen worktop
- ☐ **D.** The kitchen sink is full of glasses
- ☐ **E.** The kitchen window has let the rain in

Q9:   GF(AC7), EA, Bψ, (2, 10, 14), (C, 13, 2)

☐ **A.** When I get paid, we will stock the fridge with better produce

☐ **B.** When we are richer, we will have more food in the cupboard

☐ **C.** If I win the lottery, there will be champagne in the fridge

☐ **D.** Rich people buy food with expensive packaging

☐ **E.** The fridge is full of rich food

Q10:   F(C, 12), AC, (14, 1), D1

☐ **A.** The loud sound of the radio wakes me up

☐ **B.** I need an alarm clock to wake up

☐ **C.** I can't get to sleep when the radio is on

☐ **D.** During the day I enjoy listening to the radio at full blast

☐ **E.** In the morning, I turn up the volume of the radio to the maximum

Q11:   F(12, 14, ψ), AC9

☐ **A.** I dim the light when I feel tired

☐ **B.** I switch the TV off when I am ready to go to bed

☐ **C.** I switch off the light before going to bed

☐ **D.** When there is nothing on TV, I fall asleep

☐ **E.** I use a torch when there is a power cut

Q12:   9, F(♣, 10, 11), B♦

☐ **A.** It is dangerous to sleep with the window closed

☐ **B.** Closing a window whilst asleep can be dangerous.

☐ **C.** I can't sleep with a mirror in the bedroom

☐ **D.** Bedroom windows are not safe

☐ **E.** I don't feel safe sleeping in a bedroom with no window

CODE		
A = Personal	1 = Sound	✪ = Smooth
B = Opposite	2 = Food	❖ = Wet
C = Increase	3 = Textile	ψ = Empty
D = Extreme	4 = Size	♣ = Closed
E = Plural	5 = Furniture	♦ = Safe
F = Circumstance	6 = Ground	♥ = Green
G = Future	7 = Wealth	• = Big
J = Accept	8 = Man	∇ = Special
K = Introduce	9 = Sleep	
L = Again	10 = Room	
M = Use	11 = Glass	
N = Regular	12 = Light	
	13 = Quality	
	14 = Container	
	15 = Heat	
	16 = Wish	

Q13: 6D❖, BC13, ♥2

A. Green vegetables rot when the soil is too wet
B. The grass is greener after heavy rains
C. Edible plants don't grow well in wet soil
D. Vegetables grow best in dry soil
E. Green plants lose their colour if the soil is too wet

Q14: (A, B•, 8), BG, DBJ, ❖2

A. My son does not like soup
B. When he was younger, my son hated soup
C. My youngest son used to hate soup
D. As a child, my son would not chew his food
E. Children don't like soup

Q15: **(BA, BG), 16, K, 2, 6**

☐ **A.** I refuse to plant vegetables in the garden
☐ **B.** Planting vegetables is not something that others would have thought about
☐ **C.** I don't enjoy gardening
☐ **D.** I wasn't the one who wanted to plant vegetables
☐ **E.** In future, I will ban all vegetables from the garden

Q16: **(K, 2, 6), C(13, ♥2)**

☐ **A.** I use fertiliser to obtain better green vegetables
☐ **B.** Fertilisers increase the quality of green plants
☐ **C.** It is essential to use fertiliser to help plants grow faster
☐ **D.** Root vegetables are tastier than green vegetables
☐ **E.** Fertilising the soil helps produce better vegetables

Q17: **AGK, (♥, 11), (∇, L, M, 14)**

☐ **A.** In future, I will need to remember to recycle green glass
☐ **B.** I will place the green glass in its dedicated recycle bin later on
☐ **C.** Recyclable green glass must be placed in its own container
☐ **D.** I reuse my green bottles as containers
☐ **E.** They will introduce green glass recycle bins for my house

Q18: **∇NAF, A8, C, A7**

☐ **A.** My husband gives me money for my birthday
☐ **B.** My husband became rich last year
☐ **C.** Divorcing my husband cost me a lot of money
☐ **D.** My son occasionally wins the lottery
☐ **E.** My husband pays me a monthly allowance

CODE		
A = Personal	1 = Sound	✪ = Smooth
B = Opposite	2 = Food	❖ = Wet
C = Increase	3 = Textile	ψ = Empty
D = Extreme	4 = Size	♣ = Closed
E = Plural	5 = Furniture	♦ = Safe
F = Circumstance	6 = Ground	♥ = Green
G = Future	7 = Wealth	● = Big
J = Accept	8 = Man	∇ = Special
K = Introduce	9 = Sleep	
L = Again	10 = Room	
M = Use	11 = Glass	
N = Regular	12 = Light	
	13 = Quality	
	14 = Container	
	15 = Heat	
	16 = Wish	

Q19:   **K, 7, (7, 14), C♦**

- A. Cash kept in a safe is secure
- B. It is best to save money
- C. I find it safer to keep my cash in a box
- D. It is safer to place your money in a bank account
- E. Keeping cash under the mattress is safe

Q20:   **F(D∇F), (3,8), BJG, (E, 16)**

- A. For personal reasons, the tailor is not fulfilling orders
- B. The dry-cleaners are exceptionally busy
- C. For some reason, men's suits are no longer in fashion
- D. Due to exceptional circumstances, the tailor is not taking any further orders
- E. Due to bankruptcy, the curtain shop is closed until further notice

Q21: **Which code would best translate the following message: "The wardrobe is too small for my clothes"?**

> **A.** A(5, 3, 14), DB•, ME3
> **B.** (5, 3, 14), B10, ME3
> **C.** (5, 3, 14), DB•, MAE3
> **D.** (5, 3, 14), DBψ
> **E.** (A, 3, 4) D• (5,3,14)

Q22: **Which code would best translate the following message: "Heavy teapots are dangerous"?**

> **A.** B12, (15,❖2, 14), D15
> **B.** B, 12, 11, 14, B♦
> **C.** • (15,❖2, 14), B♦
> **D.** B12, (15,❖2, 14), B♦
> **E.** M (15,❖2, 14), B♦

Q23: **Which would be the most useful <u>two additional codes</u> to convey this message: "My wife recycles glass jars as flowerpots"?**

> **A.** Recycle
> **B.** Pots
> **C.** Ornamental
> **D.** Spouse
> **E.** Organic

Q24: **Which would be the most useful <u>two additional codes</u> to convey this message: "Babies' clothes must be washed at low temperature"?**

> **A.** Necessity
> **B.** Low
> **C.** Clean
> **D.** Clothes
> **E.** Child

CODE		
A = Personal	1 = Sound	✪ = Smooth
B = Opposite	2 = Food	❖ = Wet
C = Increase	3 = Textile	ψ = Empty
D = Extreme	4 = Size	♣ = Closed
E = Plural	5 = Furniture	♦ = Safe
F = Circumstance	6 = Ground	♥ = Green
G = Future	7 = Wealth	● = Big
J = Accept	8 = Man	∇ = Special
K = Introduce	9 = Sleep	
L = Again	10 = Room	
M = Use	11 = Glass	
N = Regular	12 = Light	
	13 = Quality	
	14 = Container	
	15 = Heat	
	16 = Wish	

Q25: **Which code would best translate the following message: "We installed poor lighting in the kitchen"?**

A. K, (B●13, 12), (2, 10)
B. (2, 10), M, (B●13, 12)
C. BG, EAK, (B●13, 12), (2, 10)
D. BG, EAM, (B●13, 12), (2, 10)
E. BG, EAK, (B♦13, 12), (2, 10)

Q26: **Which would be the most useful <u>two additional codes</u> to convey this message: "Money and happiness don't go together"?**

A. Money
B. Life
C. Negative
D. Compatible
E. Large

354

MOCK EXAM

ANSWERS

MOCK EXAM QUANTITATIVE REASONING ANSWERS

MOCK QR 1/10 – Bottling It Up

Q1.1 – d: 25%
The ratio of the 2009 price over the 2008 price is 39/52, i.e. 75%. The discount is therefore of 25%.

Q1.2 – a: £180.33
The undiscounted cost of all three red wine cases in 2009 is 40 + 33 +33 = £106. Applying a discount of 13% gives 0.87 x £106 = £92.22.

The undiscounted cost of all three white wine cases in 2009 is 39 + 24 + 36 = £99. Applying a discount of 11% gives 0.89 x £99 = £88.11.

Total cost = 92.22 + 88.11 = £180.33

Q1.3 – a: Option 1
The quickest way to approach this problem is to calculate the savings made for each category (12 x bottle price MINUS case price) and then work out the savings for the different options:

	Case price (A)	Bottle price (B)	Saving (12 B – A)
White Gold Medal Winner 2007	39	6.50	39.00
White mixed case	24	4	24.00
Red mixed case	33	5.50	33.00
Classic White Selection	36	6	36.00
Classic Red Selection	33	4.40	19.80

The answer is therefore the White Gold Medal Winner 2007 i.e. Option 1.

Q1.4 – a: 3/8
The cost of 12 bottles of Classic red selection purchased on a "per bottle" basis is 12 x 4.40 = £52.80. The saving made is therefore 52.80 – 33 = £19.80.

Expressed as a percentage of the total "per bottle" price, this gives £19.80 / £52.80 = 0.375. Since this is not easily expressed as a fraction, you can try the different solutions offered and find the appropriate one, which is 3/8.

MOCK QR 2/10 – Waste Management

Q2.1 – e: 450kg
We are told in the text that, in 2002, the average weight of glass thrown away in 2002 was 54kg. We also know from the 2002 pie chart that this represents 12% of the total waste per inhabitant. Therefore the total waste was 54/0.12 = 450kg.

Q2.2 – d: 20.8%
The weight of paper and cardboard for 1982 and 1992 are 125kg and 151kg respectively. The ratio is 151/125 = 1.208, hence an increase of 20.8% from 1982 to 1992.

Q2.3 – c: 1.45%
There are two ways of calculating this: the long way and the quick way:

The long (but most intuitive) way
We first need to calculate the total recycled weight, which must be done category by category. We know from Question 4.1 that the total amount of waste per individual was 450kg, therefore the total amount of waste across the whole population was 450 x 8700 = 3,915,000kg.

Recycled weight of paper & cardboard:
30% x 3,915,000 x 57.31% = 673,105.95kg

Recycled weight of organic elements:
25% x 3,915,000 x 80% = 783,000kg

Recycled weight of glass:
12% x 3,915,000 x 80% = 375,840kg

Recycled weight of plastic:
10% x 3,915,000 x 22% = 86,130kg

Recycled weight of metal:
6% x 3,915,000 x 80% = 187,920kg

Recycled weight of textile:
2% x 3,915,000 x 40% = 31,320kg

Recycled weight for others:
15% x 3,915,000 x 5% = 29,362.50kg

Total weight = 2,166,678.45kg

Proportion of textile = 31320 / 2,166,678.45= 1.45%

The quick way
Since we are only calculating a ratio, we do not actually need to calculate individual quantities. The ratio can be calculated as follows (using percentage values instead of fractions):

(2 x 40) / (30x57.31 + 25x80 + 12x80 + 10x22 + 6x80 + 2x40 + 15x5)
=80 / 5,534.3 = 1.45%

When a calculation seems complicated or long-winded, it is often worthwhile to take a step back to find ways to cut the time down. In this case, the long way may well take over 5 minutes to work out (not withstanding the risk of error) whereas the quick way could be done in a minute or less. Given that the first two questions are relatively quick, this would enable candidates to remain well within the time limit.

Q2.4 – b: 195,750
The total amount of organic waste is 25% x 8700 inhabitants x 450kg (see question 1) = 978,750kg.

20% of organic elements are non-recyclable (since 80% are recyclable), i.e. 195,750kg.

MOCK QR 3/10 – The Big Freeze

Q3.1 – c: – 40
We have C = (F – 32) x 5 / 9 and we want C = F.
Therefore C = (C – 32) x 5 / 9, i.e. C = – 40.

You can also get to the answer simply by calculating (F – 32 x 5/9) for all the options on offer until you find the one which works i.e.:

(– 50 – 32) x 5/9 = – 45.55 (not equal to 50 and therefore does not work)
(– 48 – 32) x 5/9 = – 44.44 (not equal to 48 and therefore does not work)
(– 40 – 32) x 5/9 = – 40 (works, since we get the same number)
This approach is just as quick.

Q3.2 – e: 671.67
We can work out the Rankine value in two stages:

1 – Convert from Celsius to Fahrenheit:
F = 9/5 C + 32 i.e. F = 212

2 – Convert from Fahrenheit to Kelvin and then from Kelvin to Rankine (note that the conversion from Kelvin to Rankine, which consists simply of multiplying by 9/5, cancels out the multiplication by 5/9 that must be done to convert from Fahrenheit to Kelvin).

Hence R = (F + 459.67) x 5/9 x 9/5, i.e. R = 212 + 459.67, i.e. 671.67.

Q3.3 – b: 98.24
The Fahrenheit value can be calculated from Kelvin as follows:
F = 9/5 x K – 459.67, i.e. F = 98.24.

Q3.4 – b: 63.32
The result can be calculated as: (15 x 1.16) x 9 / 5 + 32, i.e. 63.32.
Note that the wording suggests that it is the Celsius value which is to be increased by 16% and not the Fahrenheit, i.e. you should first add the increase and then convert.

MOCK QR 4/10 – Running Wild

Q4.1 – b: 8 mins
The quick way to get to the answer is to spot that the mother is going twice as fast as Skippy and therefore will catch up with him in half the time that it took him to get to the point where he stopped. Since it took Skippy 16 minutes to get to his destination, the mother will take 8 minutes to catch up with him.

If you used the longer approach of calculating distances, you will have calculated the following:

Distance at which Skippy stopped = 1.2 x 16/60 = 0.32 km
Time that it will take the mother to catch up = 0.32 / 2.4 = 0.1333333
Multiplying by 60 to express the result in minutes gives 8 mins

Q4.2 – d: 51 seconds
There are two ways of working this out:

The long way
After 25 seconds, Skippy will have travelled 25x20cm=500cm (5m).
At the time Skippy stops, his mother will have travelled 25x50cm=1250cm (12.5m).

The distance that she has to travel to catch up with Skippy is:
33m + 5m – 12.5m = 25.5m (i.e. the total length of the circuit + the distance Skippy has travelled minus what she has already travelled). Since she travels at a speed of 50cm per second, the time it will take her to travel is: 25.5 / 0.50 = 51 seconds.

The shorter way
After 25 seconds, Skippy will have travelled 25x20 = 5m.
When she catches up with him, his mother will therefore have travelled a total of 38m (33 metres to go round + the 5 metres he has done), which, at a pace of 50cm per seconds, will take her 76s. Deducting from this the first 25 seconds which we are told to ignore gives a time of 51 seconds.

Note: 76s is the total amount of time that she will have travelled from the start in order to catch up with him. The question is, however, related to the amount of time that she will take to catch up with him from the time of his immobilisation (i.e. 25 seconds less).

Q4.3 – c: 284 jumps

Clearly, the fastest way to get to the end is to jump with both feet at a pace of 70cm per jump. The maximum number of 70cm jumps that he can do without overshooting the target is the integral part of 198/0.7, i.e. 282.

282 jumps with both feet will achieve a distance of 282 x 0.70m = 197.4m, leaving 60cm still to go. The smallest number of jumps in which this can be achieved is two (one with the left foot, and one with the right foot, 40cm and 20cm respectively). The total minimum number of jumps is therefore 282 + 2 = 284.

Q4.4 – a: 656.25

This question can be resolved without doing any calculation. Indeed, we know that the distance separating them is 1,500m, which gives a half-way mark of 750m. We know that the father goes faster than the mother; therefore, at the time they meet, he will have walked more than 750m and she will have walked less than 750m. We are asked to calculate the distance that the mother has walked. Since Answer a is the only answer which is lower than 750m, then it has to be the correct answer.

If you want to calculate the result, it can be done as follows:

The father normally travels 1500m in 20 minutes. This makes his normal speed 4.5 km/h and therefore the mother's speed 7/9 x 4.5 = 3.5 km/h.

If we call 'M' the meeting point and 'D' the distance, MB, we are looking for:

we know that when they meet they will have travelled for the same amount of time and therefore D / 3.5 = (1.5km – D) / 4.5.

This gives:
4.5 x D = 3.5 x (1.5 – D) i.e. 8 x D = 5.35. Hence D = 0.65625km, i.e. 656.25m.

MOCK QR 5/10 – Fruity Harvest

Q5.1 – c: 2004
The sales figures for Apricots Category A were as follows:

2002: 404 x 0.75 = 303.00
2003: 73 x 1.05 = 76.65
2004: 513 x 0.60 = 307.80
2005: 417 x 0.70 = 291.90
2006: 114 x 0.95 = 108.30

The answer is therefore 2004.

Q5.2 – a: Apricots Category A
It is possible to reduce the amount of calculations involved by looking at the table briefly. A brief glance at the table will show that Nectarines cannot be the most profitable crop since their production is much lower than the production of apricots and the sales price is not that much higher. We can therefore content ourselves with calculating the income from Apricots.

Cat A: 404 x 750 + 73 x 1050 + 513 x 600 + 417 x 700 + 114 x 950 = 1.087m.
Cat B: 300 x 850 + 52 x 1200 + 354 x 750 + 312 x 800 + 57 x 1150 = 0.898m.

Hence Apricots Category A is the category with the highest income across the five years.

Q5.3 – b: £251,050
Income for 2003 = 73x1050 + 52x1200 + 64x1150 + 35x1250 = £256,400.
Projected income = 256,400 x 1.40 (40% increase) = £358,960
Cost of nets: 110 lines / 2 x 654ft x £3 = £107,910
Hence profit = £358,960 – 107,910 = £251,050

Q5.4 – a: 95,950
114 tons of Cat A apricots produce 65% x 114 = 74.1 tons of nectar.
57 tons of Cat B apricots produce 72% x 57 = 41.04 tons of nectar.
Total nectar production = 115.14 tonnes, 0r 115,140kg. This occupies a volume of 115,140 / 1.2 = 95,950 litres.

MOCK QR 6/10 – Sweet Music

Q6.1 – e: 2,856
If we call P the number of Violintown inhabitants, the total number of in-habitants can be calculated as follows:
$1508 + (P + 56) + 386 + 1456 + 3 \times 386 + P = 10,276$.
This gives us $2 \times P + 4,564 = 10,276$, i.e. $P = 2,856$.

Q6.2 – b: 1.75%
In 2005 the cost was £58,650 for 215 pupils, giving an average cost per pupil of £272.79.

In 2006, the costs were 2.7% higher for 217 pupils, giving an average of $58,650 \times 1.027 / 217 = £277.57$.

The increase in the average expenditure was therefore $277.57 / 272.79 = 1.0175$, i.e. 1.75%.

Q6.3 – e: £4,965
In 2005, there were a total of 215 pupils. Violintown's share of the costs was therefore: $37 / 215 \times 58,650 = £10,093.26$.

In 2006, Violintown shared half the costs equally with another village and therefore was liable for a quarter of the 2006 costs. Hence, Violintown's 2006 share of the costs was $1/4 \times 58,650 \times 1.027 = £15,058.39$.

Increase in costs = £4,965.13.

Q6.4 – d: 2%
The new total population would be $10,276 + 1,724 = 12,000$.
The number of pupils would be $217 + 23 = 240$. Hence the proportion of the population which studies at the school would be $240 / 12,000 = 0.02$ i.e. 2%

MOCK QR 7/10 – It Rings a Bell

Q7.1 – d: £155
Tariff 4 includes 700 minutes (covering calls to the Green network only) and 250 texts (covering texts to all networks). Therefore his telephone bill for that month would be as follows:

- Monthly fee: £35
- 300 minutes to Green network: included
- 300 minutes to H_2O network: Not included – would be charged at 40p per minute i.e. a total of £120
- Total of 250 texts: included.

Hence the total bill would be £155.

Q7.2 – e: Tariff E
His usage corresponds to 630 minutes and 450 texts. Looking at the options proposed:

- Tariff 3 would be £35 but he would need to pay for an additional 30 minutes at 15p each i.e. an extra cost of £4.50. Total £39.50

- Tariff 4 (also £35) would cover all his 630 minutes but would only cover 250 texts out of the 450 texts he expects to use (a shortfall of 200 texts). Therefore he would be liable for an additional £20. Total £55.

- Tariff C (£25) would result in having to pay for an additional 330 minutes, i.e. £99 extra. Total: £124.

- Tariff D (£30) would cover the minutes and all but 50 of the messages i.e. an extra cost of £6. Total £36.

- Tariff E (£35) would cover everything.

Q7.3 – e: 817 min
Since both tariffs include the same number of texts, the move becomes worthwhile when the cost of Tariff E including any additional minutes becomes greater than the basic cost of Tariff F, which is £40.

Tariff F will become better than Tariff E when the cost of the additional minutes is greater than £5. The additional cost of 1 minute is 30p. Therefore he will need to speak for 5 / 0.3 = 16.67 minutes, which represents the cut-off point. He would therefore need to speak for an additional 17 minutes on top of the allowance of 800 minutes i.e. a total of 817 minutes.

Q7.4 – b: 800
Tarifff 6 has a monthly fee of £55. This leaves £450 - £55 = £395 for the cost of calls (texts are not charged separately under this tariff).

Out of the calls he made, 220 + 280 + 1000 + 500 = 2000 minutes are on the Green network, with the first 1500 minutes being included in the monthly fee. There the 500 additional minutes will be charged, at a cost of 500 x 15p per minute i.e. a total of £75.

This then leaves £395 - £75 = £320 for calls made to John. Minutes spent calling the H_2O network are charged at a rate of 40p per minute. The time spent calling John was therefore 320 / 0.40 = 800 minutes.

MOCK QR 8/10 – Reward Scheme

Q8.1 – b: 5 vouchers
During the course of the quarter he will have accumulated the following points:

- Electricity: 4 points
- Grocery: 1,100 points
- Wine: 141 points
- Stationery: 15 points

Total: 1,260 points. He will receive 1 voucher for every 250 points and therefore will receive a total of 5 vouchers (with 10 points leftover).

Q8.2 – e: £47,500
570 miles are equivalent to 570 / 30 = 19 vouchers. These can be acquired by gaining 19 x 250 = 4750 points. The Electricity Company gives 1 point for each £10 spent; therefore he will need to spend £47,500.

Q8.3 – b: £375
The smallest amount needed will be obtained from the shop which provides the highest ratio of points per pound. The PS Petrol Station is the only shop which actually provides more than 1 point per pound spent (4 points per £3 spent).

To obtain a £5 discount (i.e. 2 vouchers), the client will need to acquire 500 points. At the PS Petrol Station, this would be acquired by spending 500 / 4 x 3 = £375.

Q8.4 – b: Flowers

30 coach miles would have come from 1 voucher, which is worth 250 points. The customer spent £1,250 to acquire those 250 points, therefore the conversion rate is £5 per point, which is the rate given by the Flower Shop.

MOCK QR 9/10 – Topping It Up

Q9.1 – a: 2

The amount of water that disappeared from the bowl was 500ml, 350ml of which would have been due to evaporation. Therefore 150ml were drunk by cats, which corresponds to the daily consumption of two cats.

Q9.2 – d: 11.34

The amount of water that she needed to replace every day in February is equal to the evaporation (30 ml) and the cats' consumption (5 x 75ml = 375 ml). Total = 405 ml x 28 days = 11,340ml or 11.34 litres.

Q9.3 – c: 20 birds

The evaporation level in July is 500ml, therefore the amount of water drunk was 1 litre. Out of that, 12 x 75ml (= 900ml) would have been drunk by cats, leaving 100ml for the birds. At a rate of 5ml per bird, this would give a total of 20 birds.

Q9.4 – e: 53.37

The average daily evaporation rate is calculated as:
(31 x 100 + 30 x 50 + 31 x 10) / (31+30+31) = 53.37 ml/day.

MOCK QR 10/10 – League Table

Q10.1 – d: 108

The percentage of 'A' Levels obtained at grade B at Rosamund was 70% - 30% = 40%. This corresponds to 0.4 x 270 = 108 'A' Levels.

Q10.2 – e: 33.59%

The percentage of non-A grades is calculated as 1–%A, i.e. 20%, 70%, 20%, 20% and 50% respectively. The average across all five schools is therefore calculated as follows:

(20%x450 + 70%x270 + 20%x380 + 20%x280 + 50%x320) / 1700

= 571 / 1700 = 33.59%

It is possible to get to the answer without any calculation as follows: the percentage of A grades is never more than 80%. Therefore the percentage of non-A grades for all schools is always more than 20%. The average will therefore be above 20%. Answer e (33.59%) is the only answer which is over 20%.

Q10.3 – d: 228
The girls represent 60% of 95 students, i.e. 57 students. We are also told that all students took the same number of 'A' Levels, i.e. everyone has taken 380 / 95 = 4 'A' Levels. This means that the girls took 4 x 57 = 228 'A' Levels.

Note that this can be calculated much more quickly by taking 60% of 380 (since everyone took the same number of 'A' Levels, the number taken by girls would simply be 60% of the total).

Q10.4 – c: 3.87
If 30 students took 1 A' Level only then the rest of the students (i.e. 105 – 30 = 75) took 320 – 30 = 290 'A' Levels between them. This gives an average of 290/75 = 3.87 'A' Levels per student.

MOCK EXAM
ABSTRACT REASONING
ANSWERS

MOCK AR1/13 – Shapes 1.5 to 5.5

Set A
The number of intersections within each shape is equal to 2.

Set B
The number of intersections within each shape is equal to 4. This can be achieved in any possible way (since the shapes include one object intersecting with two others, or one object intersecting with one other, or two sets of two objects intersecting with one another).

Answers
Shape 1.1: Neither. No intersection.
Shape 1.2: Set B
Shape 1.3: Neither. 6 intersections.
Shape 1.4: Neither. No intersection.
Shape 1.5: Neither. 6 intersections.

Comments
Visually, it is relatively easy to determine that all sets have intersecting objects. It is therefore a fair bet that the number of intersections will play a role. Other questions that you should have asked yourself to check possible relationships (other than the basic ones) include:

- Are the intersections between similar objects (e.g. always a triangle intersecting with a circle)? This is not the case here.

- Is there a link with the number of some of the objects (particularly for Set B, where there are many similar objects within one shape (e.g. 2 circles, 3 squares, 2 moons, 2 pentagons))? There does not seem to be a pattern here.

MOCK AR2/13 – Shapes 2.1 to 2.5

Set A
Each shape has two objects which are the same (e.g. 2 moons, 2 triangles, etc.). If there is one circle within the shape then the two objects in question are of the same size. If there are two circles within a shape then the two objects in question are of different sizes.

Set B
Set B is the reverse relationship, i.e. one circle means that the other two similar objects are of different sizes. The presence of two circles means that the other two similar objects are of the same size.

Answers
Shape 2.1: Neither. Three similar objects instead of the two required.
Shape 2.2: Neither. Only one other object.
Shape 2.3: Set B
Shape 2.4: Set A
Shape 2.5: Neither. Three similar objects instead of the two required.

Comments
The presence of circles in all shapes can be ascertained easily at a glance. Looking at the other non-circular objects, one can see that they are of a similar shape but sometimes vary in size. This should be sufficient to prompt you to investigate a relationship. Other possible relationships that you would need to investigate include:

- Whether there is a link with some of the objects overlapping (e.g. whether objects which have the same size overlap). This is not the case here.

- Whether the position of the objects matters. They look fairly random in this case.

Please note that the relationships could be much harder to ascertain if the sets contained some distracting features such as additional objects which would have little to do with the final outcome.

MOCK AR3/13 – Shapes 3.1 to 3.5

Set A: All shapes contain 10 arrowheads.
Set B: All shapes contain 7 arrowheads.

Answers
Shape 3.1: Set A
Shape 3.2: Set A
Shape 3.3: Neither. 12 arrowheads.
Shape 3.4: Neither. 8 arrowheads.
Shape 3.5: Set A

Comments
Other relationships you would need to investigate include:

- Is there a relationship between the number of double arrows and the number of single arrows (e.g. one is a multiple of the other, or one is equal to the other plus a constant)? There is no relationship here.

- Does the location of some or all of the arrows matter? For example, in Set A, four out of the six have an arrow pointing to the right at the top of each shape. But since it only appears in four of the shapes, it cannot be taken as part of any relationship.

- Does the orientation of the double arrows matter, i.e. are they all vertical or horizontal? This is not the case here.

MOCK AR4/13 – Shapes 4.1 to 4.5

Both sets contain diagrams that can be folded to make 3-dimensional boxes all having faces of the same shape.

Set A: contains sets that make boxes that are missing one side.
Set B: contains sets that make boxes with all sides complete.

Answer
Shape 4.1: Neither
Shape 4.2: Neither
Shape 4.3: Neither
Shape 4.4: Set A

Shape 4.5: Neither. When the object is folded it does make a pyramid with one side missing but the missing side is square, not triangular.

Comments
When an exercise contains shapes with squares presented in blocks in such a manner, the relationship usually revolves around the fact they can be folded to make a specific object (e.g. a cube, a pyramid, etc.).

MOCK AR5/13 – Shapes 5.1 to 5.5

Set A:
The number of white circles is the square of the number of black circles (e.g. 4 whites and 2 blacks; 16 whites and 4 blacks).

Set B:
The number of white circles is the cube of the number of black circles (e.g. 8 whites and 2 blacks; 64 whites and 4 blacks).

Answers
Shape 5.1: Set A
Shape 5.2: Set A
Shape 5.3: Neither. 2 blacks, 5 whites.
Shape 5.4: Neither. 2 blacks, 6 whites.
Shape 5.5: Set B

Comments
Some of the shapes contain many circles and it could take time to count them all. Consequently, some candidates may be put off counting them. It is always worth doing a quick count on some of the less crowded shapes to see if a pattern can be established. If, after counting a sample of shapes, you detect a possible pattern, you can then move on to counting some of the more crowded shapes. The counting for the most crowded shape (first one in Set B) is made easier by the layout (7 by 7 square).

Other relationships you may want to investigate include:

- Does the position of the circles within each shape matter? Some of the shapes have the same number of white/black circles (e.g. in Set A, two shapes have 2 blacks and 4 whites), which indicates that the position of the circles within the shape is likely to be irrelevant.

- Does the relative position of black circles in relation to white circles matter? The type of relationship that you are looking for may be as follows: "if there are 2 black circles then the white squares are above the line that links them", "if there are 3 black circles, the white squares are contained within the triangle drawn by linking them", "if there are 4 black circles, the white circles are contained within the parallelogram drawn by linking them", etc. This is not the case here.

MOCK AR6/13 – Shapes 6.1 to 6.5

Set A:
Each large object contains one <u>black</u> object only, which is of the same type, e.g. a single small black square within a large square object; a single small black triangle within a large triangle.

Set B:
Each large object contains one <u>white</u> object only, which is of the same type, e.g. a single small white square within a large square object; a single small white triangle within a large triangle.

Note that in both sets the number of small objects which are of the opposite colour is irrelevant.

Answers
Shape 6.1: Neither. No small object is uniquely black or white.
Shape 6.2: Neither. No small object is uniquely black or white.
Shape 6.3: Set A
Shape 6.4: Neither. Two objects of a unique colour but not matching the large object.
Shape 6.5: Set A. (The uniquely coloured small object is a black circle, which matches the large circle. The fact that there is also a white circle is irrelevant.)

Comments
Other relationships that you would need to investigate include:

- Is the number of objects of the opposite colour (i.e. white for Set A and black for Set B) linked to the object in the unique colour? For example, it could be that the small black object is a triangle (i.e. has three sides) then there are three white objects. This is not the case here.

- Does the total number of objects equal the number of sides of the big object e.g. a large square contains 4 objects whilst a large triangle contains 3 objects? This does not apply here.

- Does the location of the small objects within the large object matter (e.g. it could be that the single coloured object is always in the same place)? This is not the case here.

MOCK AR7/13 – Shapes 7.1 to 7.5

Set A:
Within each shape the number of dots on each domino is the same, e.g. in the first shape, the two dominoes each have 7 dots (4+3 and 3+4).

Set B:
Within each shape, the number of dots on each of the two diagonals adds up to the same number, i.e. the sum of the top dots on the first domino plus the bottom dots on the second domino equals the sum of bottom dots on the first domino plus the top dots on the second. In the first shape of the set, the total along the diagonals is 7 (4+3 and 2+5).

Note that the total varies between the different shapes and therefore the actual number of dots within one shape is not relevant.

Answers

Shape 7.1:   Set A
Shape 7.2:   Neither
Shape 7.3:   Neither
Shape 7.4:   Set A
Shape 7.5:   Neither

Comments
Shapes centred around dominoes will most often be related through the number of dots they contain. Try the following relationships:

- Adding or multiplying all dots in the shape.
- Adding or multiplying the dots on each independent domino.
- Adding or multiplying the dots on the diagonals.
- Adding or multiplying the dots horizontally.

Other possible relationships include:

- The number of dots in the top half is greater or lower than the number of dots in the bottom half.

- The number of dots in the top half is a multiple of the number of dots in the lower half (e.g. double or triple).

- Odd versus even number of dots.

MOCK AR8/13 – Shapes 8.1 to 8.5

Set A: The number of small <u>white</u> objects is equal to the number of sides of the large object.

Set B: The number of small <u>black</u> objects is equal to the number of sides of the large object.

Answers
Shape 8.1: Set A
Shape 8.2: Set B
Shape 8.3: Set B
Shape 8.4: Neither. We would require 3 small objects of the same colour.
Shape 8:5: Neither. We would need only 1 small object of a given colour.

Comments
When shapes all contain a large object then these objects are the primary driver for the relationships. Relationships that you should particularly be looking for include:

- Are there smaller objects of the same type as the large object (e.g. if the large object is a square, are there smaller squares too)? This is not always the case here.

- Is the relationship linked to the number of sides? This is the case here.

- Is the relationship linked to the number of objects outside/inside the shape? This is not the case here.

MOCK AR9/13 – Shapes 9.1 to 9.5

Both sets contain at least one triangle, one circle and one square, with one of the three objects being duplicated. This creates a pair of objects and two "twins".

Set A: There is no rule about the colour of the objects. However, the twins must face each other and not lie in adjacent quarters of the shape.

Set B: Adjacent quarters must not contain objects of the same colour (i.e. we always have two black objects facing each other and two white objects facing each other). The twins must lie adjacent to each other and therefore must be of differing colour.

Answers
Shape 9.1:   Set A
Shape 9:2:   Neither. There are only 2 types of object in the shape.
Shape 9.3:   Neither. The twins follow the right relationship for Set B but we would also need to have a black square instead of a white square opposite the black circle.
Shape 9.4:   Neither. There are only 2 types of object in the shape.
Shape 9.5:   Neither. There are only 2 types of object in the shape.

Comments
The separation in four quadrants makes it easier to identify the relationships. If you identify quickly that the shapes only contain three possible objects: circle, square and triangle, then the only possible relationships are as follows:

- The object in one specific quadrant is always of the same colour (not the case here).
- Objects facing each other are either of the same type or of the same colour, or both (this is the case here for Set A).
- Objects adjacent to each other are either of the same type or of the same colour, or both (this is the case here for Set B).
- If an object of a specific type is of a certain colour, then another object of a specific type is of the same colour or the opposite colour, e.g. if the triangle is black then the circle is also black (this is not the case here).

MOCK AR10/13 – Shapes 10.1 to 10.5

The relationships are linked to the direction of the arrows and the number and type of objects within each shape. All arrows are vertical and all objects (other than the arrow) are white. The size and position of the objects do not matter.

In both sets, when the arrow points upwards, the number of objects (excluding the arrow) is even. When the arrow points downwards, the number of objects (excluding the arrow) is odd.

Set A:
- When the arrow points downwards, all other objects are different.
- When the arrow points upwards, all objects are of the same type, though not necessarily the actual same shape or the same size (e.g. four triangles of different natures).

Set B:
- When the arrow points upwards, all other objects are different.
- When the arrow points downwards, all objects are of the same type, though not necessarily the actual same shape or the same size (e.g. three different types of ovals, five different pentagons, or 7 diamonds).

Answers
Shape 10.1: Set A
Shape 10.2: Neither. A downward pointing arrow requires an odd number of objects to belong to either set.
Shape 10.3: Neither. 8 similar objects plus a different object.
Shape 10.4: Set B
Shape 10.5: Set A

Comments
Your eyes are naturally drawn towards large objects. Do not spend time worrying about them if you can see that only some shapes have large objects (e.g. 2nd shape, left column, Set A). You will waste valuable time.

Similarly, your eye will be drawn to shapes which contain objects of a similar nature (e.g. 7 diamonds of equal size in Set B, 5 pentagons in Set B). This may well be relevant, but it may also be a sizeable distractor which will waste your time.

You may well find that you cannot take your mind away from such shape; if it is the case, go back to basics and start counting objects and sides. Look out also for the nature of the sides (i.e. curved v. straight).

MOCK AR11/13 – Shapes 11.1 to 11.5

The relationship is linked to the nature of the overlapping area between the two objects (note that it is the not the shape of the object itself which matters but the shape of the overlapping area).

Set A: There is always one black object and one white object. If the overlapping area only contains straight edges then it is filled with vertical lines. If the overlapping area contains at least one curved edge then the black object is always on top of the white object.

Set B: There is always one black object and one white object. If the overlapping area contains at least one curved edge then the white object is always on top of the black object. It the overlapping area contains only straight edges then the white object is always underneath the black object.

Shape 11.1: Neither. The overlapping area only contains straight edges. It should therefore be striped in order to belong to Set A. To belong to Set B, it would require having the white object underneath the black object.

Shape 11.2: Set B

Shape 11.3: Set B

Shape 11.4: Neither. The overlapping area is a circle and therefore has curved edges. It is shaded. In Set A, only overlapping areas with straight edges are shaded. There is no shading in Set B).

Shape 11.5: Set A

MOCK AR12/13 – Shapes 12.1 to 12.5

Set A: All black pieces can be put together to form exactly the white object.

Set B: All white pieces can be put together to form a reduced-sized replica of the black object.

Answers
Shape 12.1: Set B
Shape 12.2: Set A
Shape 12.3: Neither
Shape 12.4: Set B
Shape 12.5: Neither

Comments
The easiest starting point when you have both large and small objects is to start counting the small objects and to see how the count relates to the other shapes. Often the count will relate to one of the following:
- Number of sides
- Number of right angles
- Number of straight or curved edges
- Number of objects with a certain feature (e.g. number of objects with right angles, number of objects of a certain colour, number of objects with a given number of sides).

When you have shapes which all contain objects with two colours, there is most often a factor that differentiates them, i.e. they are rarely used as distractors. Possible differences include:
- Number of sides (i.e. either a fixed number or an odd/even number)
- Curved v. straight edges
- Symmetrical v. asymmetrical
- Right angles v. non-right angles
- Angles less than or more than 180 degrees.

Comments
Relationships which involve putting objects together to make up another object tend to be the hardest to spot. Some people are very good at spotting such relationships visually whilst others don't find it so natural. Look out for the shapes that present better clues than others (for example, the first two shapes in Set A's first column which are clearer than the others in that respect). Similarly, the 3rd shape in Set B's left column (the two stars) may provide a valuable insight.

You will often find that the clues come from 2 or 3 shapes. Once you have picked up on a possible relationship, you can then test it on the other shapes in order to either confirm or reject it.

MOCK AR13/13 – Shapes 13.1 to 13.5

Every shape contains three objects, two of which overlap and one of which is stand-alone.

Set A: The number of sides of the stand-alone object equals the number of intersections between the other two objects.

Set B: The number of sides of the stand-alone object equals the number of intersections between the other two objects + 1.

Answers
Shape 13.1: Set A
Shape 13.2: Set A
Shape 13.3: Neither. There are 8 intersections, with the stand-alone object having 5 sides.
Shape 13.4: Neither. Only 2 intersections, with the stand-alone object having 4 sides.
Shape 13.5: Set B

Comments
The fact that two of the three objects overlap should be easy to notice. Your reflex should be to count the number of intersections. This will usually lead you to the answer.

MOCK EXAM VERBAL REASONING ANSWERS

MOCK VR1/11 – Christmas Repeats

Q1.1 – CAN'T TELL
We know that 16% of BBC1's programmes were repeats. We know that 60% of Channel 5's programmes were repeats. Without knowing how many programmes both broadcasters showed, it is not possible to compare the actual number of repeats.

Q1.2 – CAN'T TELL
Using the same logic as for Q1, we know that the proportion of repeats has not changed. However, without knowing the actual number of programmes in both years, we cannot comment on the actual number of repeats.

Q1.3 – CAN'T TELL
The text presents no link between the decrease in viewing share suffered by terrestrial channels and the increase in repeats. It just states the facts. In fact there is no clear evidence as to whether viewers want to see repeats or not other than a survey by the broadcasters themselves.

Q1.4 – TRUE
We are told that Channel 4's share fell by more than 11% to 8.7%. Therefore its share in 2006 was over 19.7%. We are also told that BBC2's share in 2006 was 11.9%. Therefore Channel 4 was more popular than BBC2 in 2006.

MOCK VR2/11 – HIV Vaccine

Q2.1 – FALSE
The text explains clearly that he hopes to develop a therapeutic vaccine, which is administered to people who are already infected and is designed to help fight the consequences of the infection. Therefore it will not stop

people being infected in the first place (this would be a preventative vaccine).

Q2.2 – TRUE
According to the last paragraph, the reservoir of the virus which sits in organs and tissues can be reactivated when treatment has stopped. Therefore until that reservoir can be eliminated, it remains a clear barrier to the eradication of the virus.

Q2.3 – CAN'T TELL
If the vaccine fails, the patient will need to revert to the combination therapy. Whilst some patients may not need therapy thereafter, some may. Therefore we cannot conclusively state that the assertion is true or false.

Q2.4 – CAN'T TELL
All we know from the text is that efforts to develop a preventative vaccine have so far been unsuccessful (and that the reservoir is an obstacle). There is nothing to suggest that a preventative vaccine is impossible.

MOCK VR3/11 – E-cigarette

Q3.1 – CAN'T TELL
It is unclear as to whether the toxicity is to the user or to those around him/her, i.e. whether any of the toxic products are contained in the vapour. All we know is that the liquid in the cigarette contains toxic substances. The vapour, we are told, contains aromatic essences. There is also uncertainty about what the final approval will depend on. The text suggests that the authorities have two main issues: toxicity but also misleading advertising claims. There is no indication as to whether the authorities are aiming to make the cigarette less toxic or whether approval will mainly be linked to more honest advertising claims. If approval depended on the removal of all toxic substances, then it would be correct to say that the e-cigarette would remove the dangers of passive smoking. However, if approval depended solely on the introduction of less misleading advertising then the toxicity would remain and therefore the dangers of passive smoking may not be removed.

Q3.2 – CAN'T TELL
We know the linalol and menthol contained in the e-cigarette can cause convulsions in the elderly, and those with epilepsy. However, it does not mean that no one else can suffer from similar effects. It would be fair to

say that young people who are not epileptic are likely to have a lower risk, but not that the e-cigarette is safe (which is a very definite statement).

Q3.3 – TRUE
Absolutely, we cannot say that this will happen, but the key to the answer is in the word "could". We know that e-cigarettes are currently being advertised as smoking-cessation devices, a claim which the health authorities are investigating. That claim is only illegal because proper approval was not sought, but it does not mean that it is factually incorrect. Whether or not e-cigarettes will eventually be used to encourage smokers to quit smoking is subject to final approval, but the use of the word "could" in the statement makes it a true claim (i.e. there is a viable possibility). If the statement were worded as "In the future, e-cigarettes WILL be used to encourage smokers to give up smoking", then the answer would be "Can't tell" because it would depend on whether approval is granted.

Q3.4 – TRUE
No licence was obtained to commercialise the product (a licence is needed because of potential toxicity and possible use for smoking cessation), therefore it is illegal to commercialise the product.

MOCK VR4/11 – NICE

Q4.1 – CAN'T TELL
The text states that "Lord Darzi has <u>recommended </u>that the approval time be reduced to 3 months" and that "NICE has been criticised for being slow to reach decisions (up to 2 years)". However, this is only a recommendation rather than fact. We therefore can't say that NICE <u>will be required</u> to make decisions in under 3 months.

Q4.2 – FALSE
The text states clearly that NICE decisions only apply to NHS treatments and that patients can access non-approved treatments if they pay for them themselves. It is therefore not correct to state that patients cannot receive treatment in the UK unless the cost is under £30,000.

Q4.3 – TRUE
The key sentence is "This means that some treatments which could add a lot of value to a patient are discounted because they are too expensive."

Q4.4 – FALSE

We are told that NICE decisions are binding and the NICE applies to the NHS only; therefore, within NICE, decisions will apply uniformly to all patients. There may be inequalities of care, for example between NHS patients (who are constrained by NICE) and private patients (who can pay for unapproved treatment themselves), but such inequalities are not taking place within the NHS.

MOCK VR5/11 – Heavy Metal

Q5.1 – FALSE

TQH is a measure of the risk posed by the wine, rather than a measure of the concentration of heavy metals. There are several clues for this:

- In the text, THQ is called a "risk evaluation index" and is actually called a "Hazard Quotient".
- We are also told that THQ analyses risk to long-term exposure to chemical pollutants; it will therefore measure the risk posed by the metals rather than their concentration.
- We are told that the scientists looked at several studies showing the quantities of metal present in the wine. That information is therefore already known. THQ is measured subsequently.

Q5.2 – TRUE

The countries are listed from best to worse. First we are told that Argentina, Brazil and Italy have the lowest concentrations; that France is not well ranked and is followed in decreasing order by Austria, Spain, Germany and Portugal; and, finally, that Hungary and Slovakia have the highest concentrations. The main difficulty with this part of the text is to determine what is meant by "decreasing order". Is it in decreasing order in terms of level of concentration, i.e. from high concentrations to low concentrations, or decreasing order from the best ranked (i.e. those with low concentration) to worst ranked (i.e. those with high concentration). Since the text first lists the best performing wines and ends with the worst performing wines, the context indicates that the countries are listed from best to worst. Hence, Portugal fares worse than Spain and therefore has a higher concentration of heavy metals.

Q5.3 – CAN'T TELL

The last paragraph suggests that not all metal may be assimilated, and in particular that rhamnogalacturonan may neutralise metallic elements. However, all these aspects are introduced as part of a debate/discussion

on the issue, and therefore nothing can be definitely asserted. Any risk is presented as potential only.

Q5.4 – FALSE
There were indeed sixteen countries involved but the scientists did not question any wine drinkers. They merely analysed studies which had been carried out previously by others.

MOCK VR6/11 – Women in Ancient Egypt

Q6.1 – CAN'T TELL
The text states that "it was perhaps unsafe for an Egyptian woman to venture far from her town alone". The use of the word "perhaps" indicates that this a speculative statement and therefore we cannot conclude whether it is true or not.

Q6.2 – CAN'T TELL
We know that two-thirds of property would be distributed between the two children. However, we are not being told whether the property is being shared equally between the two children (for example, it could be that the elder gets a bigger share). There is also ambiguity about the meaning of "property". The text refers to two-thirds of the "community property" whereas the question only refers to "property" in general.

Q6.3 – CAN'T TELL
We know that there were a hundred female doctors in Ancient Egypt (though we are not told whether these doctors lived at the same time). We also know that there were few women in administrative positions, though we are not told how many.

Q6.4 – FALSE
The concept of fairness is not defined in the text but we know from the first paragraph that there were inequalities between the different classes. Therefore, although we cannot conclude from the text whether Egypt was a fair society, we do know that it was not classless. Therefore the assertion (which combines both terms with an "and") is false.

MOCK VR7/11 – The Eye of the World

Q7.1 – FALSE
Hubble is not earth-bound.

Q7.2 – CAN'T TELL
The fact that Hubble, which has a smaller mirror than the Chilean telescopes, produces pictures of better quality cannot be generalised since we are comparing telescopes that are being used in different environments. To be able to answer this question conclusively, we would need to have data which compared mirror sizes in similar circumstances (e.g. two mirrors of different sizes at the same altitude in space or in the Chilean desert).

Q7.3 – CAN'T TELL
We are not told anything about the quality of images before the repairs, when Hubble was "short-sighted". In the absence of any knowledge on the extent of the damage, we cannot conclude either way.

Q7.4 – TRUE
The text says that "some of its instruments are over a decade old", which suggests that others are less than 10 years old. In turn, this means that newer instruments were added during some of the service missions (or that older instruments were replaced).

MOCK VR8/11 – Green Fly

Q8.1 – FALSE
Although ANZ used a mix of kerosene and biofuel, Virgin Airlines did a trial flight with palm oil and coconut oil only. Whether this can be done in the long term is another matter; but the text suggests that this flight actually took place and, therefore, that planes can fly on 100% biofuel.

Q8.2 – CAN'T TELL
We are told that jatropha can be grown on very dry soil but nothing in the text indicates that it could not be grown on soil normally used for food.

Q8.3 – CAN'T TELL
We know from the text that the use of first generation biofuels encouraged deforestation. We conclude from this that locals would cut trees down to plant corn, soya, rapeseed or other suitable plants. If jatropha were to be used, since it can be grown on very dry soil, we can anticipate that locals would try to use naturally dry areas and would not need to cut trees down. However, unless we can be reassured that jatropha cannot be grown on the type of soil that forests occupy, there is no reason to assume that lo-

cals would not cut down trees to grow it. There is just a lesser chance that they might.

We know that it is non-negotiable condition that the use of biofuels should not interfere with food cultures; however this is not the same as saying that it should not lead to deforestation.

Q8.4 – CAN'T TELL
The text does not address the "green" issue. For example, we are not told anything about what the oil-refining process involves, how much carbon planes will release when the fuel is being burnt, or anything else for that matter. "Being green" is also not one of the criteria used by ANZ.

MOCK VR9/11 – Unwanted Goods

Q9.1 – FALSE
Both bullet points make it clear that the rules apply whatever the reason for returning the teapot. Therefore the level of refund does not depend on the reason given but only on the criteria listed in the bullet points (e.g. level of admin fees, damage to the teapot, time elapsed since receipt of the teapot).

Q9.2 – TRUE
Mrs Ackroyd did not receive any refund. This could happen only in three circumstances:
- Mrs Ackroyd cancelled within the 7 or 14-day period following receipt of the teapot and returned the teapot damaged. But she is being thanked at the end of the letter for sending the teapot back undamaged; therefore this is not a valid assumption to make.
- Mrs Ackroyd cancelled within the 7 or 14-day period following receipt of the teapot and incurred a credit card and/or admin fee which was greater than the cost of the teapot; however, we are told that this is not the shop's policy.
- Mrs Ackroyd cancelled more than 14 full days after receiving the teapot. If she received the teapot on 4 April then this means she has complained on or after 19 April.

Q9.3 – FALSE
Based on the text, if someone cancelled an order from this shop within 7 days of receipt of a teapot and sent the teapot back undamaged, then,

since they would not incur any card or administration charges, they would get a full refund.

Q9.4 – FALSE
8 July is 7 full days after the date of order (1 July). The date from which the 7 days are counted is the date the item is <u>received</u>, not the date of the order. Therefore it is incorrect to say that the "retailer has no obligation to grant any refund if the order is cancelled after 8 July". For example, if an item was received on 10 July then the customer would get a full refund provided they cancelled on or before 17 July.

MOCK VR10/11 – The Veggie Diet

Q10.1 – CAN'T TELL
The text tells us that a B12 deficiency may cause anaemia ("vegans... risk developing a Vitamin B12 deficiency and therefore anaemia"). This does not mean that all anaemia can be solely caused by a B12 deficiency. We therefore cannot conclude that a patient with anaemia will also have a Vitamin B12 deficiency. All we can conclude from this sentence is that someone who does not have anaemia cannot have a Vitamin B12 deficiency.

Q10.2 – FALSE
Vitamin B12 is exclusively present in foods of animal origin (first sentence of second paragraph). Therefore cress, which is a vegetal, cannot be a source of Vitamin B12. It is a source of calcium though. However, since the assertion asks us to comment on calcium and Vitamin B12 together, then it is false.

Q10.3 – CAN'T TELL
We know that vegetarians tend to smoke less than non-vegetarians; however, we would need to understand the precise link between smoking and lung cancer to draw a conclusion (and, remember, we cannot use our external knowledge). In any case, even if we knew for certain from the text that smoking increased the risk of lung cancer, the statement would not necessarily be true. For example, it could be that vegetarians are exposed to other factors which lead to lung cancer and to which non-vegetarians may not necessarily be exposed (e.g. some pesticides, asbestos, etc.). The only way we could conclude that this statement is true would be if: (i) we were being told so; or (ii) we knew that smoking increases the risk of

lung cancer and was the main cause. Finally, there is a reduction of some cancers in vegetarians but we don't know which cancers.

Q10.4 – CAN'T TELL
This question plays on the differentiation between percentages and numbers. Intuitively, one would think that, if vegetarians have a low rate of obesity compared to non-vegetarians, they would make up a minority in the obese group. However, this is not necessarily so as it depends on the relative size of the groups. For example, imagine a world where we have 1000 vegetarians, 10% of whom (i.e. 100) are obese, and 100 non-vegetarians, 50% of whom (i.e. 50) are obese. This would confirm what the text says about a lower proportion of vegetarians being obese (10% v. 50%) but when looking at the obese population, they would make up 100 out of the 150 obese people, i.e. two-thirds. So unless we know the relative sizes of the two groups, we cannot conclude either way.

MOCK VR11/11 – Pole Position

Q11.1 – FALSE
This position is correct as far as the Academy of Medicine is concerned; however, the CNRS report, we are told, does not bear judgement on the negative effects of radio frequencies. So the report does not state that there is no danger.

Q11.2 – FALSE
Since the exposure is maximal at a distance of 280 metres, it can't be linear and therefore can't be proportionate to the distance.

Q11.3 – CAN'T TELL
The text does not address the issue of rural areas, but only those relating to urban areas or areas immediately adjoining urban areas.

Q11.4 – TRUE
In fact, from the text, we can even say that it is higher than 1.5 V/m.

MOCK EXAM
DECISION ANALYSIS
ANSWERS

Q1 – MOCK DA
A: The duvet is too big.

3, 5, 9 = Textile, (Sleep, Furniture)
D4 = Extreme Size

This could be literally translated as "The bed sheet is of extreme size". Answer A, although not a perfect match, is the closest. Looking at the alternatives:

Answer B: My bed takes up too much space
The coded message does not contain the notion of "Personal" so the resulting translation should remain generic. In addition, this translation introduces the notion of "bed" rather than "Textile".

Answer C: Your sleeping bag is too big for me
This introduces "I" and "you", neither of which are present in any form within the coded message.

Answer D: The bed sheet is too large for me
The notion of "me" is not present in the coded message. Answer A is closer in that regard.

Answer E: My tailor is rich
The original message does not mention any person or notion of wealth, only of textile and size.

Q2 – MOCK DA
C: Your towel is not dry

BA = Opposite Personal
❖10, 3 = Wet Room, Textile
❖ = Wet

This code contains several notions:

- A wet room, which could be a bathroom, a sauna or any other room which has a link to water.
- A textile from that room, e.g. a towel, shower curtain, which must be wet.
- The fact that the textile is not mine.

Accordingly, Answer C is the most appropriate answer. Looking at the alternatives:

Answer A: My shower curtain is dry
This uses "My", which contradicts the phrase "Opposite Personal".

Answer B: Your soap is wet
This does not use the notion of "Textile".

Answer D: The bathroom floor needs mopping up
The mop could be considered as textile; however, the coded message does not imply any sense of action. Also, the message does not contain anything that would remotely relate to a "floor" or to a "need". Finally, the phrase "Opposite Personal" is not being used.

Answer E: Your face cloth needs to dry
This adds the notion of "face", which could be okay if there was no other, more general, option. However, this introduces the notion of "need", which the original message does not contain.

Q3 – MOCK DA
C: The bathroom window is frosted

11 = Glass
❖10 = Wet Room
B❂ = Opposite Smooth

This could be literally interpreted as "The glass in the bathroom is not smooth", which is close to Answer C. Looking at the other answers:

Answer A: The shower screen is missing
The use of "shower screen" is appropriate. However, the coded message mentions "Opposite Smooth" which cannot be interpreted as "missing".

Answer B: The bath taps are dirty

The word "dirty" would be an appropriate translation of "Opposite Smooth"; however, the answer makes no use of the concept of "glass".

Answer D: The shaving mirror is old

"Shaving mirror" is a possible translation for "Glass, Wet Room", although the mention of shaving is superfluous and therefore makes it less appropriate than an answer such as Answer C which is more generic. The word "old" is not a good translation for "smooth" unless one talks about something which wrinkles.

Answer E: Your bathroom light is flickering

"Bathroom light" is a loose translation of "Glass, Wet Room". In any case, the use of "your" introduces an individual perspective which is not contained in the coded message.

Q4 – MOCK DA
E: My bedroom curtains block out the sun

A, 9, 10, 3	= Personal, Sleep Room, Textile
DBC	= Extreme Opposite Increase
12	= Light

This could be literally interpreted as: "My textile in the bedroom drastically decreases the light", which fits Answer E closely. Looking at the alternatives:

Answer A: My bedroom carpet is getting dirty

"Bedroom carpet" fits the concept of "Sleep Room Textile" well and this answer is translating "Extreme Opposite Increase Light" as "Getting Dirty". Getting dirty would fit the concept of becoming darker, i.e. less light; however, this does not allow for the notion of "Extreme".

Answer B: My blanket is too thin

This does not convey the notion of "Opposite Increase". It merely states the fact that it is thin (with the "too" conveying the concept of "Extreme").

Answer C: The bedroom rug is wearing out

The concept of "Light" could indeed be used to describe something which is becoming lighter as in losing weight and therefore the notion of wearing is relevant. However, in this message "Light" is decreasing and therefore

"Opposite Increase Light" would mean actually getting heavier, which is not the case here. In any case, the coded message contains "Personal", which is not being used in this answer.

Answer D: The bedroom curtains are very pale

Similarly to Answer C, "Opposite Increase Light" should be translated by "getting darker" rather than being pale. This answer is therefore the wrong way round, does not convey the notion of "Opposite Increase" and does not use "Personal".

Q5 – MOCK DA
D: The window cleaner gets paid more when it rains

8, 11✪   = Man, Glass Smooth
C7   = Increase Wealth
F❖   = Circumstance Wet

This could translate as "The man with smooth glass (or the man who smoothes glass) increases wealth when it is wet", which seems to fit Answer D. Looking at the alternatives:

Answer A: The plumber wears expensive glasses

This does not make use of "Smooth" or "Increase".

Answer B: Cleaning windows costs more after heavy rain

There is no notion of "heaviness" in the coded message, which would typically be translated as "Extreme", only of "wetness". In addition, this translation does not use "Man" and therefore is a looser interpretation of the coded message, which Answer D adheres to more closely.

Answer C: The glazier charges more in the winter

"Glazier" could be a loose interpretation of "Man Glass Smooth" since strictly speaking a glazier installs windows rather than smoothes them, but in any case this interpretation talks about winter which is a very loose interpretation of "Circumstance Wet" and would be best described as "Circumstance Cold".

Answer E: Men who wear glasses clean them more often when it rains. The first bracket contains the words "Man Glass Smooth" and therefore one would expect those three words to be together in the translation. The phrase "Men who wear glasses" ignores the "Smooth" part of

the code, which is used a bit later with the concept of cleaning. There is also no notion of "increasing wealth" in this translation.

Q6 – MOCK DA
B: I sleep better with the light on

A   = Personal
C, 13, 9   = Increase, Quality, Sleep
F, 12   = Circumstance, Light

This could translate as "I increase the quality of sleep when there is light", which fits Answer B. Looking at the alternatives:

Answer A: I sleep little but well
Here, the code word "Light" is translated as little and defines the sleep. In the coded message, however, the word "Light" is used as a circumstance.

Answer C: It is better to sleep with the light on
This translation ignores the "Personal".

Answer D: I sleep more in the summer
"Light" does not necessarily equate to summer, though if the other options were equally vague, this translation would stand. In any case, this translation does not mention quality of sleep but only quantity.

Answer E: In the summer I have a good siesta
This does not use the notion of "Increase". Also, as for D, "Light" does not necessarily equate to "summer".

Q7 – MOCK DA
A: My neighbour's constant noise keeps me awake

8   = Man
BA10   = Opposite Personal Room
D1   = Extreme Sound
AB9   = Personal Opposite Sleep

This could be literally translated as "The man opposite my room makes an awful lot of noise (or very loud noises) and I can't sleep", which fits Answer A more closely than the others. Looking at the alternatives:

Answer B: My husband's snoring stops me from sleeping
This does not use the concept of "Opposite Room". In addition, the "Personal" is linked to the room rather than the man. Husband could be best described as "Personal Man".

Answer C: Men find it difficult to sleep in my bedroom
This does not use the "Opposite Room" part of the code. In addition, this translation does not mention "Sound" anywhere.

Answer D: Sleeping can be hard when you have neighbours who party all the time.
The code does not contain the notion of "party", only of "Extreme noise". In addition, the word "Man" is used in the singular whereas "neighbours" is a plural generalisation. Finally, the coded message uses "Personal" twice, which is not reflected in this translation.

Answer E: I don't sleep well when my neighbour is too noisy
This is not a bad translation but it is slightly less appropriate than Answer A. This notion of not sleeping well is linked to quality rather than "Opposite Sleep", i.e. lack of sleep. Also, the coded message is more general. Answer E suggests that it is only when the neighbour is noisy that the person is not sleeping well, whereas the coded message implies that the neighbour is generally noisy and that is why the person is not sleeping well. Answer E would have been more appropriate if the code had contained the code F for "Circumstance".

Q8 – MOCK DA
D: The kitchen sink is full of glasses

2, 10, ❖5	= Food, Room, Wet Furniture
Bψ	= Opposite Empty
E(11,14)	= Plural (Glass, Container)

This could be literally translated as "The wet furniture in the food room (i.e. kitchen or lounge) full several glass containers" which does not mean much since there is no verb to guide us as to what the relationship between the three components of the sentence is. The absence of a verb points us towards the direction of a simple "implicit" verb such as "is" or "has", which would make Answer D suitable. Looking at the other options:

Answer A: The glasses cabinet has watermarks
This does not make use of the notion of "full". Nor does it use the notion of "Food Room" since we are not told where the glasses cabinet is located.

Answer B: The kitchen tap is clogged up with limescale
Kitchen taps are a sensible translation for "Food, Room, Wet Furniture" but the word "limescale" bears no relationship to the notion of "Plural Glass Container".

Answer C: I spilt water on the kitchen worktop
The coded message does not contain the notion of "Personal". This translation also ignores the notion of "Glass Container".

Answer E: The kitchen window has let the rain in
What this translation says is that the kitchen furniture is wet because of the window. It does therefore contain the notion of "Food Room Wet Furniture"; however, in the code, these four words are together, i.e. there is no concept of the furniture becoming wet, but more a sense of belonging. Finally, this option does not use the notion of "full".

Q9 – MOCK DA
A: When I get paid, we will stock the fridge with better produce

GF(AC7)	= Future Circumstance (Personal, Increase, Wealth)
EA, Bψ	= Plural Personal, Opposite Empty
2, 10, 14	= Food, Room, Container
C, 13, 2	= Increase, Quality, Food

This can be literally interpreted as "When I increase my wealth in the future, we will fill a cupboard/container in the food room (i.e. kitchen or dining room) with food of better quality", which matches Answer A. Looking at the alternatives:

Answer B: When we are richer, we will have more food in the cupboard.
This is not a bad translation; however, it mentions "when we are richer" when the coded message does not associate the notion of "Plural" with "Personal" when it deals with the "Wealth". Also, this answer talks of having more food rather than better quality food (the code is explicit on the notion of "Quality").

Answer C: If I win the lottery, there will be champagne in the fridge

Winning the lottery is a substantial extrapolation on the concept of "Increase Wealth", though it would be acceptable if there were no better alternatives. This answer also equates "champagne" with "Quality", which is very subjective. Finally, champagne is not really something that could be labelled as food. In this sense, Answer A is more generic and therefore more appropriate.

Answer D: Rich people buy food with expensive packaging

This answer does not use the concept of "Personal".

Answer E: The fridge is full of rich food

This does make use of the concepts of "Personal" or "Quality".

Comments

Answer A is not an exact or literal translation of the code. For example, the coded message has the concept of "Increase Wealth", which is translated in the answer as "When I get paid". The link is questionable in the sense that getting paid is just one possible interpretation of "Increase Wealth", though not necessarily the most intuitive. However, on balance, Answer A provides the closest fit considering all other factors since it makes use of all the concepts introduced by the code and is more generic than Answer C.

Q10 – MOCK DA
E: In the morning I turn up the volume of the radio to the maximum

$F(C, 12)$	= Circumstance (Increase, Light)
AC	= Personal Increase
14, 1	= Container Sound
D1	= Extreme Sound

This could be literally interpreted as "When the light increases, I increase the radio to an extreme sound", for which Answer E is a good fit. Looking at the alternatives:

Answer A: The loud sound of the radio wakes me up

All the elements are there (e.g. waking up is a possible, though loose, translation of "Increase Light"), but not quite in the right order. For example, "Increase Light" is marked as a circumstance and not the effect of

noise. It should therefore be translated as "When I wake up" for this sentence to work best.

Answer B: I need an alarm clock to wake up
The code does not contain the notion of "need". Also, this answer does not make use of the concept of "Extreme Sound".

Answer C: I can't get to sleep when the radio is on
This uses the fact that the radio is on as a circumstance whereas the coded message is "Increase Light" as a circumstance. The concept of "Increase Light" is not being used and certainly cannot be translated by "can't get to sleep". Finally, this does not use the concept of "Extreme Sound".

Answer D: During the day, I enjoy listening to the radio at full blast
The coded message does not contain the notions of "enjoy" or "listening". Also "During the day" does use the concept of "Light" but not of "Increase". The concept of "morning" used in Answer E is closer since morning can be considered as the period when daylight increases.

Q11 – MOCK DA
D: When there is nothing on TV, I fall asleep

F(12, 14, ψ) = Circumstance (Light, Container, Empty)

AC9 = Personal Increase Sleep

This could be literally interpreted as "When the light container is empty, I increase my sleep", which Answer D is a possible match for if we interpret "Light Container" as TV. Note that in Answer D, the terms "Increase Sleep" are translated by the concept of falling asleep, i.e. an increased state of sleepiness. Although not necessarily intuitive, the translation is acceptable as it conveys the notion of increase.

To determine whether this is the closest match available, we need to look at the other options:

Answer A: I dim the light when I feel tired
In the coded message, the circumstance is linked to the light and the action to the sleep. In Answer A, we have the opposite, i.e. the circumstance is the "feeling tired" and the action is in "dimming the light".

Answer B: I switch the TV off when I am ready to go to bed

Similarly to Answer A, the switching off of the TV should be the circumstance, not the action taken. Also, "I am ready to go to bed" does not convey in any sense the idea of "Increase Sleep", whereas in Answer D "falling asleep" implies an increased state of sleepiness. Finally, the coded message uses the concept of the TV being empty as a circumstance rather than a consequence of wanting to go to bed.

Answer C: I switch off the light before going to bed

The code for "Circumstance" relates to "Light Container Empty", not to "Personal Increase Sleep".

Answer E: I use a torch when there is a power cut

This answer does not use the concept of "Sleep".

Q12 – MOCK DA
A: It is dangerous to sleep with the window closed

9 = Sleep

F(♣, 10, 11) = Circumstance (Closed, Room, Glass)

B♦ = Opposite Safe

This could be interpreted as "Sleep when the window of the room is closed is not safe", which matches answer A if we assume that the term "window" is the translation of "Room Glass".

Note that the phrase "Closed Room Glass" can be interpreted in many ways e.g. there is a mirror in a closed room". We therefore need to look at the alternatives to ensure that there are no other answers which are closer.

Answer B: Closing a window whilst asleep can be dangerous

This answer gathers all the right elements but not in the right place. In the coded message "Closed Room Glass" is the circumstance rather than the action and it is the sleeping which is dangerous rather than the action of closing the window. Finally, the answer introduces a notion of possibility with the word "can", which is not present in the coded message.

Answer C: I can't sleep with a mirror in the bedroom

The answer does not address the concept of "safety" or of "Closed", and introduces the notion of "I", which does not feature in the coded message.

Answer A is therefore closer. Answer C would be valid/closer if it read "It is dangerous to sleep in a closed room with a mirror".

Answer D: Bedroom windows are not safe

The concept of "bedroom" comes from the combination of "Sleep" and "Room". However, these are not together within the message. This answer also ignores the notion of "Closed". Finally, windows are plural in this answer, but not in the code.

Answer E: I don't feel safe sleeping in a bedroom with no window

The coded messages talks about a closed window rather than the absence of one. Also, this answer uses "I", a notion which is not contained within the coded message.

Q13 – MOCK DA
A: Green vegetables rot when the soil is too wet

6D❖	= Ground Extreme Wet
BC13	= Opposite Increase Quality
♥2	= Green Food

This can be literally interpreted as "An extremely wet ground decreases the quality of green food". This is close to Answer A. Looking at the alternatives:

Answer B: The grass is greener after heavy rains

This does not use the notion of "Opposite Increased Quality" or "Ground". There is also a question mark over whether "Green food" can be interpreted as "grass", though this makes some sense if we understand it as food for animals.

Answer C: Edible plants don't grow well in wet soil

This does not use the notion of "Extreme".

Answer D: Vegetables grow best in dry soil

This is a double negation of the coded message but cannot be deduced so easily, i.e. the fact that vegetables lose quality in an extremely wet soil does not mean that they would grow well in a dry soil.

Answer E: Green plants lose their colour if the soil is too wet

Losing colour is not the same as losing quality.

Q14 – MOCK DA
B: When he was younger, my son hated soup

A, B●, 8   = Personal, Opposite Big, Man
BG   = Opposite Future
DBJ   = Extreme Opposite Accept
❖2   = Wet Food

This can be literally interpreted as "My small man, in the past, categorically refused wet food", which Answer B suits well. Looking at the alternatives:

Answer A: My son does not like soup
This does not use the notion of "Opposite Future", i.e. past.

Answer C: My youngest son used to hate soup
This applies the code "Extreme" to the concept of "Opposite Big". The coded message only conveys that the person is not big, not that they are the smallest (or youngest).

Answer D: As a child, my son would not chew his food
This construction of the sentence is a close match to the coded message. However, the idea of "not chewing food" is not equivalent to rejecting liquid food.

Answer E: Children don't like soup
This does not use the notions of "Opposite Future" and "Personal".

Q15 – MOCK DA
D: I wasn't the one who wanted to plant green vegetables

BA, BG   = Opposite Personal, Opposite Future
16, K, 2, 6 = Wish, Introduce, Food, Ground

This could be literally interpreted as: "Not me, in the past, wished to introduce food in the ground", which matches Answer D. Looking at the other options:

Answer A: I refuse to plant vegetables in the garden
Although the word "garden" could be seen as a suitable translation for "Ground" within the context of this sentence, Answer A is not suitable because it does not make use of the "Opposite Future" concept.

Answer B: Planting vegetables is not something that others would have thought about.
This is interpreting the coded message the wrong way round. "Not me" can indeed be interpreted as "Others" but we would then have "Others wished to plant vegetables", which is totally different to the meaning conveyed by Answer B. In addition, the word "thought" has a different meaning to the word "Wish" present in the coded message. Not thinking about it would mean they would not have considered it, whereas not wishing it would mean that they had considered it but rejected it.

Answer C: I don't enjoy gardening
This answer does not make use of the "Opposite Future" concept, and in fact does not mention anything about introducing food either. In addition, the negative in the coded message is linked to "Personal" rather than to the "Introduce".

Answer E: In future, I will ban all vegetables from the garden
This explicitly mentions "In future", when the coded message actually states the opposite. In addition, the negative in the coded message relates to "Personal" and not to "Introduce".

Q16 – MOCK DA
E: Fertilising the soil helps produce better vegetables

K, 2, 6   = Introduce, Food, Ground
C   = Increase
13, ♥2   = Quality, Green Food

This can be literally interpreted as "Introducing food into the ground increases the quality of green food", which matches Answer E. Looking at the alternatives:

Answer A: I use fertiliser to obtain better green vegetables
This answer is a close contender, but it introduced a notion of "I" which is not found in the coded message.

401

Answer B: Fertilisers increase the quality of green plants

"Green plants" are not necessarily food and therefore the translation is slightly inaccurate. In addition, the answer does not make use of "Introduce" although, to some extent, it is implied that the fertilisers will increase quality if introduced into the ground (and not when left in the box).

Answer C: It is essential to use fertiliser to help plants grow faster

The coded message does not make any reference to speed of growth, only to the quality of the final product. In addition, there is no notion of "essential" in the coded message.

Answer D: Root vegetables are tastier than green vegetables

This answer interprets "Food Ground" as root vegetables, which is a sensible translation; however it ignores the "Introduce". This answer also mentions taste whereas the coded message simply mentions quality.

Q17 – MOCK DA
B: I will place the green glass in its dedicated recycle bin later on

AGK   = Personal Future Introduce

♥, 11   = Green Glass

∇, L, M, 14 = Special, Again, Use, Container

This can be literally interpreted as "I will introduce green glass in a special container for using again", i.e. a good match for Answer B. Looking at the alternatives:

Answer A: In future, I will need to remember to recycle green glass

Although this introduces the notion of recycling, it does not explicitly talk about a special container being used. In addition, this introduces a notion of "remember" which is not in the coded message.

Answer C: Recyclable green glass must be placed in its own container. This answer does not use the notions of "Personal" or "Future".

Answer D: I reuse my green bottles as containers

This does not use the notion of "Introduce" or "Future".

Answer E: They will introduce green glass recycle bins for my house

The coded message does not mention any external influence ("They") or any house.

Q18 – MOCK DA
A: My husband gives me money for my birthday

∇NAF	= Special Regular Personal Circumstance
A8	= Personal Man
C	= Increase
A7	= Personal Wealth

This can be literally translated as "On a special regular personal circumstance (e.g. maybe a birthday, an anniversary, etc.), my personal man (e.g. a husband, son, etc.) increases personal wealth (could be his or mine). This fits Answer A well. Looking at the alternatives:

Answer B: My husband became rich last year
This is not a "Regular Personal Circumstance", only a one-off.

Answer C: Divorcing my husband cost me a lot of money
This is not a regular event and conveys badly the notion of increasing personal wealth (it could be that the loss of money was in legal fees and not necessarily money going to the husband).

Answer D: My son occasionally wins the lottery
This does not use the notion of "Regular".

Answer E: My husband pays me a monthly allowance
This does not constitute a "Special" circumstance.

Q19 – MOCK DA
D: It is safer to place your money in a bank account

K, 7	= Introduce, Wealth
7, 14	= Wealth, Container
C♦	= Increase Safe

This can be literally interpreted as "Introducing money into a money container (e.g. bank, safe, savings account, etc.) is safer". This closely matches Answer D. Looking at the alternatives:

Answer A: Cash kept in a safe is secure
It is debatable as to whether "secure" is equivalent to "Safe", but, even if you accept that this is the case, the answer does not use the "Increase".

Answer B: It is best to save money
Saving money is not necessarily the same as placing it into a "container" e.g. one can save money simply by spending less rather than physically placing money somewhere. Also the word "best" is very loose and does not necessarily imply safety.

Answer C: I find it safer to keep my cash in a box
The word "box" is not very specific. The coded message does not just say "Container", it says "Wealth Container". One would therefore expect the mention of some form of saving instrument. In addition, this interpretation contains the word "I" whereas the coded message is generic and not personal.

Answer E: Keeping cash under the mattress is safe
Similarly to Answer C, a mattress might just about be considered a "Container" in this context, but not a "Wealth Container". In addition, the answer ignores "Increase".

Q20 – MOCK DA
D: Due to exceptional circumstances, the tailor is not taking any further orders

F(D∇F)	= Circumstance (Extreme Special Circumstance)
3, 8	= Textile, Man
BJG	= Opposite Accept Future
E, 16	= Plural Wish

This can be literally interpreted as "Since there are extremely special circumstances, the textile man will not accept wishes", which is closely matched by Answer D. Looking at the alternatives:

Answer A: For personal reasons, the tailor is not fulfilling orders
This mentions personal reasons which are not mentioned in the coded message. The coded message is more explicit, talking about "Extreme Special Circumstance", which do not have to be personal. In addition, not fulfilling orders is not the same as not accepting further orders; indeed this implies he is not fulfilling current orders.

Answer B: The dry-cleaners are exceptionally busy
This makes no reference to not accepting wishes/orders/requests in future.

Answer C: For some reason, men's suits are no longer in fashion
The mention of "some reason" should be enough to allow you to discount this answer as a viable option since it does not contain any notion of "Extreme" or "Special". In addition, the code is clear that it is the wishes that are not accepted in future, rather than the clothes.

Answer E: Due to bankruptcy, the curtain shop is closed until further notice. Bankruptcy is a very narrow interpretation of "Extreme Special Circumstance" and would be best coded using "Wealth". Answer D is more generic and therefore more in line with the coded message. In addition, this answer mentions a shop when the coded message mentions a "Man". Also, being closed until further notice is not the most appropriate interpretation of "not accepting wishes in future" in that it is too extreme.

Q21 – MOCK DA
C: (5, 3, 14), DB●, MAE3

Answer C translates as (Furniture, Textile, Container), Extreme Opposite Big, Use Personal Plural Textile, which matches closely the message that needs translating.

Other answers would translate as follows:

Answer A: Personal (Furniture, Textile, Container) Extreme Opposite Big, Use Plural Textile introduces the notion of "Personal" before the wardrobe and would therefore translates as "My wardrobe is too small for clothes".

Answer B: (Furniture, Textile, Container), Opposite Room, Use Plural Textile can be translated as "The wardrobe has no room for clothes", which is not quite the same as saying that it is too small. Answer C is closer to the message to be coded.

Answer D: (Furniture, Textile, Container), Extreme Opposite Empty essentially means "The wardrobe is full", which is not to say that it is too small.

Answer E: (Personal, Textile, Size) Extreme Big (Furniture, Textile, Size) literally means "The size of my clothes is very big for my wardrobe" which is the other way round compared to the message.

Q22 – MOCK DA
D: B12, (15, ❖2, 14), B◆

Answer D translates as Opposite Light, (Heat Wet Food Container), Opposite Safe, requiring an interpretation of "Wet Food" as Liquid and the whole middle bracket (Heat Wet Food Container) as "teapot". Although this seems slightly distant from the message that we are trying to convey, this is the best translation amongst the codes proposed.

Looking at the other answers:

Answer A: *Opposite Light, (Heat Wet Food Container), Extreme Heat.*
This only says that heavy teapots are very hot, not that they are dangerous.

Answer B: Opposite, Light, Glass, Container, Opposite Safe.
This codes "teapot" as "Glass Container", which is not as close a code as "Heat Wet Food Container", which conveys a sense of hot liquid and not just a container.

Answer C: Big (Heat, Wet Food, Container), Opposite Safe.
This codes "Heavy" as "Big", which is not as good as the "Opposite Light" used in other answers.

Answer E: Use (Heat, Wet Food, Container), Opposite Safe.
This introduces the code for "Use", which makes sense, but does not address the "Heavy" part of the message.

Q23 – MOCK DA
C: Ornamental & D: Spouse

The word "Recycle" can be coded easily as "Use Again".
"Pots" can be coded as "Plural Container".
The word "Organic" is not really required to code "flower" since we already have "Green".

The two words required are
- "Spouse", since to code "wife" properly, we would need to write something like: "Personal Special Opposite Man", which is convoluted.
- "Ornamental", which goes well with Green to describe "flowers".

Q24 – MOCK DA
A: Necessity & C: Clean

The word "Low" can be coded easily as "Opposite Big", which would work well when associated with the word "Heat".

The word "Clothes" can be coded easily as "Plural Textile".

The word "Child" can be translated as "Personal Special Opposite Big Man".

However, there is nothing at all in the code to translate "must", hence we need Answer A: "Necessity". There also is nothing in the code to convey the notion of "wash". Having Answer C "Clean" would therefore be useful.

Q25 – MOCK DA
C: BG, EAK, (B•13, 12), (2, 10)

Answer C translates as "Opposite Future, Plural Personal Introduce, (Opposite Big Quality Light) (Food Room)", which is a close match to the components found in the message to code. Looking at the other answers:

Answer A: Introduce, (Opposite Big Quality, Light), (Food, Room)
This does not code the notion of "We", which is coded with "Plural Personal" in Answer C. This also does not contain any notion of "past".

Answer B: (Food, Room), Use, (Opposite Big Quality, Light)
This could translate as "The kitchen uses poor lighting". Although the idea is there, this is not quite what the message to code is conveying and this code is also missing the "Personal" touch and the notion of "past".

Answer D: Opposite Future, Plural Personal Use, (Opposite Big Quality), (Food, Room) translates into "We used poor lighting in the kitchen" and does not convey the notion of "install".

Answer E: Opposite Future, Plural Personal Introduce, (Opposite Safe Quality, Light), (Food, Room) introduces the concept of "safety" which is not contained in the message to code.

Q26 – MOCK DA
B: Life & D: Compatible

In this sentence, there are essentially three concepts that we need to code:

Concept 1: Money, which can be translated by "Wealth". This means that Answer A (Money) is not required.

Concept 2: Happiness, which can be translated by "Big Quality Life" or simply "Quality Life" since there is no specific code for it. Consequently, we would require Answer B: "Life".

Concept 3: Going together, for which there is no code at present. However, Answer D "Compatible" would suit this concept well.

Looking at the other answers:

- "Negative" is not required since we already have "Opposite".
- "Large" is not required since we already have "Big".

MOCK EXAM
MARKING SCHEDULES

MARKING SCHEDULE

For each of the questions, write your score in reference to the maximum mark in the box provided. You should score your answers as follows:
- Zero if you gave the wrong answer or failed to answer at all.
- Max mark if you answered correctly.

QUANTITATIVE REASONING			
Question	Answer	Max Mark	Your Mark
1.1	d	20	
1.2	a	25	
1.3	a	25	
1.4	a	20	
2.1	e	20	
2.2	d	20	
2.3	c	30	
2.4	b	20	
3.1	c	25	
3.2	e	25	
3.3	b	20	
3.4	b	20	
4.1	b	20	
4.2	d	30	
4.3	c	20	
4.4	a	25	
5.1	c	25	
5.2	a	25	
5.3	b	25	
5.4	a	20	
6.1	e	20	
6.2	b	20	
6.3	e	25	
6.4	d	20	
7.1	d	25	
7.2	e	25	
7.3	e	25	
7.4	b	25	

Question	Answer	Max Mark	Your Mark
8.1	b	20	
8.2	e	20	
8.3	b	25	
8.4	b	20	
9.1	a	20	
9.2	d	20	
9.3	c	20	
9.4	e	20	
10.1	d	20	
10.2	e	25	
10.3	d	20	
10.4	c	25	
TOTAL		900	

ABSTRACT REASONING			
Shape	Answer	Max Mark	Your Mark
1.1	Neither	13	
1.2	B	13	
1.3	Neither	13	
1.4	Neither	13	
1.5	Neither	13	
2.1	Neither	13	
2.2	Neither	13	
2.3	B	13	
2.4	A	13	
2.5	Neither	13	
3.1	A	14	
3.2	A	14	
3.3	Neither	14	
3.4	Neither	14	
3.5	A	14	
4.1	Neither	14	
4.2	Neither	14	
4.3	Neither	14	
4.4	A	14	
4.5	Neither	14	
5.1	A	14	

Shape	Answer	Max Mark	Your Mark
5.2	A	14	
5.3	Neither	14	
5.4	Neither	14	
5.5	B	14	
6.1	Neither	14	
6.2	Neither	14	
6.3	A	14	
6.4	Neither	14	
6.5	A	14	
7.1	A	14	
7.2	Neither	14	
7.3	Neither	14	
7.4	A	14	
7.5	Neither	14	
8.1	A	14	
8.2	B	14	
8.3	B	14	
8.4	Neither	14	
8.5	Neither	14	
9.1	A	14	
9.2	Neither	14	
9.3	Neither	14	
9.4	Neither	14	
9.5	Neither	14	
10.1	A	14	
10.2	Neither	14	
10.3	Neither	14	
10.4	B	14	
10.5	A	14	
11.1	Neither	14	
11.2	B	14	
11.3	B	14	
11.4	Neither	14	
11.5	A	14	
12.1	B	14	
12.2	A	14	
12.3	Neither	14	
12.4	B	14	

Shape	Answer	Max Mark	Your Mark
12.5	Neither	14	
13.1	A	14	
13.2	A	14	
13.3	Neither	14	
13.4	Neither	14	
13.5	B	14	
TOTAL		900	

VERBAL REASONING			
Question	Answer	Max Mark	Your Mark
1.1	Can't tell	20.5	
1.2	Can't tell	20	
1.3	Can't tell	20.5	
1.4	True	20.5	
2.1	False	20.5	
2.2	True	20.5	
2.3	Can't tell	20.5	
2.4	Can't tell	20.5	
3.1	Can't tell	20.5	
3.2	Can't tell	20.5	
3.3	True	20.5	
3.4	True	20.5	
4.1	Can't tell	20.5	
4.2	False	20.5	
4.3	True	20.5	
4.4	False	20.5	
5.1	False	20.5	
5.2	True	20.5	
5.3	Can't tell	20.5	
5.4	False	20.5	
6.1	Can't tell	20.5	
6.2	Can't tell	20.5	
6.3	Can't tell	20.5	
6.4	False	20.5	
7.1	False	20	
7.2	Can't tell	20.5	
7.3	Can't tell	20.5	
7.4	True	20.5	

Question	Answer	Max Mark	Your Mark
8.1	False	20.5	
8.2	Can't tell	20.5	
8.3	Can't tell	20.5	
8.4	Can't tell	20.5	
9.1	False	20	
9.2	True	20.5	
9.3	False	20.5	
9.4	False	20.5	
10.1	Can't tell	20.5	
10.2	False	20.5	
10.3	Can't tell	20.5	
10.4	Can't tell	20.5	
11.1	False	20.5	
11.2	False	20	
11.3	Can't tell	20.5	
11.4	True	20.5	
TOTAL		900	

DECISION ANALYSIS			
Question	Answer	Max Mark	Your Mark
1	A	35	
2	C	35	
3	C	35	
4	E	35	
5	D	35	
6	B	35	
7	A	35	
8	D	35	
9	A	35	
10	E	35	
11	D	35	
12	A	35	
13	A	35	
14	B	35	
15	D	35	
16	E	35	
17	B	35	
18	A	35	

Question	Answer	Max Mark	Your Mark
19	D	35	
20	D	35	
21	C	34.5	
22	D	34.5	
23 Word 1	C	16	
23 Word 2	D	16	
24 Word 1	A	16	
24 Word 2	C	16	
25	C	35	
26 Word 1	B	16	
26 Word 2	D	16	
TOTAL		900	

SUMMARY TABLE

QUANTITATIVE REASONING SCORE	/ 900
ABSTRACT REASONING SCORE	/900
VERBAL REASONING SCORE	/ 900
DECISION ANALYSIS SCORE	/ 900
TOTAL SCORE	/ 3600
AVERAGE SCORE (= TOTAL SCORE / 4)	/ 900

PREPARE FOR YOUR MEDICAL SCHOOL INTERVIEW WITH ISC MEDICAL

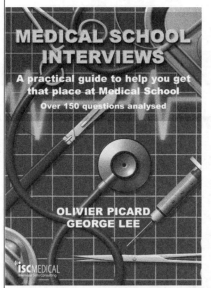
Visit our website for all your medical school application needs including resources to write a winning personal statement and small-group courses to prepare for your medical school interview.

Book through our website: www.iscmedical.co.uk or call us on 0845 226 9487 for more details.